Ego Functions in Schizophrenics, Neurotics, and Normals: A Systematic Study of
Conceptual, Diagnostic, and Therapeutic Aspects
*by Leopold Bellak, Marvin Hurvich, and Helen A. Gediman*

Innovative Treatment Methods in Psychopathology
*edited by Karen S. Calhoun, Henry E. Adams, and Kevin M. Mitchell*

The Changing School Scene: Challenge to Psychology
*by Leah Gold Fein*

Troubled Children: Their Families, Schools, and Treatments
*by Leonore R. Love and Jacques W. Kaswan*

Research Strategies in Psychotherapy
*by Edward S. Bordin*

The Volunteer Subject
*by Robert Rosenthal and Ralph L. Rosnow*

Innovations in Client-Centered Therapy
*by David A. Wexler and Laura North Rice*

The Rorschach: A Comprehensive System
*by John E. Exner*

Theory and Practice in Behavior Therapy
*by Aubrey J. Yates*

Principles of Psychotherapy
*by Irving B. Weiner*

Psychoactive Drugs and Social Judgment: Theory and Research
*edited by Kenneth Hammond and C. R. B. Joyce*

Clinical Methods in Psychology
*edited by Irving B. Weiner*

PSYCHOACTIVE DRUGS
AND SOCIAL JUDGMENT

# PSYCHOACTIVE DRUGS AND SOCIAL JUDGMENT:
## THEORY AND RESEARCH

*Edited by*

KENNETH R. HAMMOND
*University of Colorado*

C. R. B. JOYCE
*CIBA-GEIGY Limited*

A WILEY-INTERSCIENCE PUBLICATION

JOHN WILEY & SONS, New York • London • Sydney • Toronto

**Library of Congress Cataloging in Publication Data**

Main entry under title:

Psychoactive drugs and social judgment.

    (Wiley series on personality processes)
    "A Wiley-Interscience publication."
    Includes bibliographies.
    1.  Psychopharmacology.  2.  Judgment.
3.  Interpersonal relations.  I.  Hammond, Kenneth R.
II.  Joyce, Charles Richard Boddington.
RC483.P77      615'.78      75-16136
ISBN 0-471-34728-0

Printed in the United States of America

10 9 8 7 6 5 4 3 2 1

# *Contributors*

RICHARD L. COOK, Institute of Behavioral Science, University of Colorado, Boulder, Colorado

JOHN S. GILLIS, Department of Psychology, Texas Tech University, Lubbock, Texas

ELLEN R. GRITZ, Brentwood Veteran's Administration Hospital, Los Angeles, California

KENNETH R. HAMMOND, Institute of Behavioral Science, University of Colorado, Boulder, Colorado

MURRAY E. JARVIK, Department of Psychiatry, University of California at Los Angeles, Los Angeles, California

C. R. B. JOYCE, Pharmaceutical Division, Clinical Research, CIBA-GEIGY Limited, Basel, Switzerland

MICHAEL K. LINDELL, BATTELLE, Human Affairs Research Center, Seattle, Washington

CARL D. MOSS, Department of Psychology, Texas Tech University, Lubbock, Texas

THOMAS R. STEWART, Institute of Behavioral Science, University of Colorado, Boulder, Colorado

DENNIS VARONOS, Department of Pharmacology, University of Athens Medical School, Athens, Greece

HART F. WEICHSELBAUM, Institute of Behavioral Science, University of Colorado, Boulder, Colorado

NICHOLAS ZACHARIADIS, Consultant Psychiatrist and Research Associate, University of Athens, Athens, Greece

RITA ZIMBELMAN, Northwest Denver Comprehensive Community Mental Health Center, Denver, Colorado

# *Series Preface*

This series of books is addressed to behavioral scientists interested in the nature of human personality. Its scope should prove pertinent to personality theorists and researchers as well as to clinicians concerned with applying an understanding of personality processes to the amelioration of emotional difficulties in living. To this end, the series provides a scholarly integration of theoretical formulations, empirical data, and practical recommendations.

Six major·aspects of studying and learning about human personality can be designated: personality therapy, personality structure and dynamics, personality development, personality assessment, personality change, and personality adjustment. In exploring these aspects of personality, the books in the series discuss a number of distinct but related subject areas: the nature and implications of various theories of personality; personality characteristics that account for consistencies and variations in human behavior; the emergence of personality processes in children and adolescents; the use of interviewing and testing procedures to evaluate individual differences in personality; efforts to modify personality styles through psychotherapy, counseling, behavior therapy, and other methods of influence; and patterns of abnormal personality functioning that impair individual competence.

IRVING B. WEINER

*Case Western Reserve University*
*Cleveland, Ohio*

# *Preface*

This book is the product of many hands. Not only does each author have his own research assistants and secretarial staff to thank for their contributions, but also the group as a whole had the benefit of the deep, personal interest of two dedicated assistants who carried out the data analysis for all the studies and, in addition, made it their business to see that the book was put together properly. Karene Will and Bertha Ramsay carried out the data analysis for each project, proofread and checked every chapter for accuracy of content and style, and made the illustrations as well. It is easy to imagine that this project could have been started without these two, but impossible to imagine that it would have been completed without them. Carol Fernandez and Amy Alsbury typed the manuscript and deserve special thanks for a difficult job done well.

We also wish to express our gratitude to the Rockefeller Foundation for offering the hospitality of its Study and Conference Center at Bellagio, Italy, to Hammond during the month of October, 1973, in order to allow him to work on the preparation of the present volume.

Professor H. J. Bein, Dr. P. Loustalot, and Professor R. Oberholzer gave their personal support as well as that of the CIBA-GEIGY Company.

We acknowledge with thanks permission granted us from the Society for the Study of Psychological Issues to reprint pages from "New Directions in the Study of Conflict Resolution," *Journal of Social Issues*, 1965, **21,** 44–66. That publication led to our first meeting and to this collaboration.

Kenneth R. Hammond
C. R. B. Joyce

*Boulder, Colorado*
*Basel, Switzerland*
*April 1975*

# Contents

*Interpersonal Conflict*

*Interpersonal Learning*

PART THREE   NEW DIRECTIONS

# Figures

PSYCHOACTIVE DRUGS
AND SOCIAL JUDGMENT

# Introduction

KENNETH R. HAMMOND and C. R. B. JOYCE

This book directs attention to a psychological theory that has enabled investigators to obtain new information about the effects of psychoactive drugs on social judgment. Thus it concerns the effects of psychoactive drugs on the cognitive process most directly implicated by social failure. The specific topics studied are *learning to improve judgment, interpersonal conflict,* and *interpersonal learning.* It was the opportunity to study the effects of psychoactive drugs on human judgment in relation to these critical aspects of social interaction that brought the present group of investigators together, and that resulted in the present volume.

Because of our belief that scientific progress comes from the continual interaction of theory, method, and data, we are explicit about the conceptual framework that sets the course for the research. In Chapter 1, Gritz and Jarvik provide a general review of studies (through 1973) concerning the effects of psychoactive drugs on social behavior. In Chapter 2, Cook narrows the discussion; he limits his review to research that has employed the methods of experimental social psychology to study the therapeutic effects of psychoactive drugs. In Chapter 3, Hammond narrows the discussion still further; he describes the theory of social judgment from which the research procedures employed in the present investigation were derived.

Part II contains the 10 empirical studies that were carried out within the conceptual framework set forth in Chapter 3. The results of these studies show that the procedures used are capable of detecting the effects of psychoactive drugs on social judgment with regard to all three topics mentioned above—particularly so in the case of persons hospitalized for mental illness. Perhaps the most important result is the one that is most evident—the social judgment of psychotic patients is impaired by the drugs most frequently used to treat them.

These results are based on coordinated experiments carried out in Greece and in

1

the United States by several investigators (pharmacologists, psychologists, computer scientists, and a psychiatric nurse) during 1971–1973. Since most of the investigators were involved in several different studies, the editors had the choice of grouping the material by topic, or by author. We chose the former method on the assumption that the reader's preference is to find studies grouped by topic rather than by author. The first chapter dealing with each topic describes in detail the procedures common to all the chapters grouped together, an arrangement that assumes that the leading chapter will be read first. Repeated description of procedures common to several studies is thus avoided.

Part III looks to research in the future. Gillis, Stewart, and Gritz describe the use of new computer technology, developed in connection with the theory of social judgment presented here, to study the judgment processes of schizophrenic patients and methadone addicts. Weichselbaum shows how one of the more important new concepts—cognitive control—provided by the theory was used to detect the deleterious effect of methadone. Stewart, Joyce, and Lindell describe the extension of the theory to another aspect of the problem of determining the effects of drugs. They show (a) that part of the problem involved in executing and interpreting the trials of all new drugs is due to differences in physicians' judgments of patients' signs and symptoms, (b) that these differences can be reduced, and (c) that the value of the treatment studied can be more sensitively estimated. In Chapter 17, Joyce and Hammond describe the implications of the previous chapters for future relations between pharmacology, sociopsychological research, and society in general.

Disparate as well as mutual interests are reflected in the two major sources of financial support for the research. The National Institute of Mental Health (NIMH) has, for a long period of time, supported research concerning social judgment, including studies involving interpersonal conflict and interpersonal learning, because competent social judgment is considered to be essential to successful participation in society. A program of research on these topics has been carried out at the Institute of Behavioral Science of the University of Colorado, with considerable support from the university as well as NIMH, for many years.

The research on the effects of psychoactive drugs on social judgment was initiated by CIBA-GEIGY, a large, international pharmaceutical company. They supported the research mainly because of the need for better methods for screening psychoactive drugs. It is common knowledge that present methods (which ordinarily involve psychiatric ratings of patients) for evaluating the effects of psychoactive drugs are less than satisfactory; both the reliability and validity of these methods leave a great deal to be desired. Because the research procedures introduced here include the advantages of experimental rigor, as well as much of the complexity of social interaction, it was hoped that the combination of rigor and social representativeness might eventually become more useful than procedures that continue to rely mainly on the mysteries of clinical judgment. It is important to note that because new procedures were being used, emphasis was placed on scrutinizing the new procedures, rather than on characterizing specific effects of specific drugs in a definitive way. That step was postponed until it was determined whether the methods used were capable of detecting at least broad effects of well-known drugs on social judgment. In our view, that has been accomplished; the possible synergism between drugs and social judgment can now be explored in a more detailed fashion.

The role of the editors was primarily that of coordinating the research. Joyce was responsible for the pharmacological side of the study; Hammond was responsible for the psychological side. Together, they are pleased to offer the work to those interested in the effects of psychoactive drugs on human judgment, as well as to those interested in the psychology of social judgment per se. This volume is the product of nearly 10 years of intercontinental collaboration between the editors, as well as between some of the investigators; an undertaking not easy to organize, to initiate or to complete—even on one continent. Our enthusiasm for what has been accomplished does not, however, blind us to the fact that what we present is merely a beginning and is, therefore, likely to suffer from the difficulties inherent in all efforts to take new directions. Whether the theory and technique should be explored further, or whether they are now ready to be used for the evaluation of psychoactive drugs, new and old, is a matter to be decided upon by the reader.

# PART ONE

# Problem: Theory: Method

Part I provides a broad background for the empirical studies that follow. First, literature on psychoactive drugs and social behavior is reviewed with the aim of offering the reader a general overview of the results of research so far. Second, the literature on the therapeutic use of psychoactive drugs is considered, with particular emphasis on studies that have employed sociopsychological methods. Third, the theory and methods intrinsic to social judgment theory are described in detail. This chapter provides the basis for the empirical work described in Part II.

# CHAPTER 1

# Psychoactive Drugs and Social Behavior

ELLEN R. GRITZ and MURRAY E. JARVIK

Since the mid-1950s there has been a tremendous growth of interest in the effects of drugs upon behavior. Two factors are largely responsible: first, the development of really useful drugs for the treatment of psychiatric disorders; second, a very marked and perhaps related increase in the use of drugs for recreational purposes (see Jarvik, 1970a; Brecher, 1972). Both kinds of widespread drug use have spurred research into the neuropharmacological mechanism of action of these agents. This has led to a greater understanding of their actions, and has also thrown some light on the disease processes they are used to treat.

Before the 1950s the pharmacological armamentarium of the psychotherapist was exceedingly limited. Sedative-hypnotic drugs were the main agents used, plus pure or impure placebos. The bromides used in the nineteenth century to sedate inpatients and to induce sleep were largely displaced in the twentieth century by barbiturates, of which phenobarbital was far and away the favorite. These drugs obviously had some effect upon the treatment of insomnia, but were also popular for the daytime sedation of anxiety and various neurotic disorders. However, there were no drugs to treat the more serious psychiatric disorders, such as psychoses or deep depressions or mania, until the clinical introduction of chlorpromazine in 1952 (see Delay, Deniker, & Harl, 1952) and of reserpine in 1954 (see Schlittler, MacPhillamy, Dorfman, Furlenmeier, Huebner, Lucas, Mueller, Schwyzer, & Saint-Andre, 1954); these drugs launched psychopharmacology as an important therapeutic field. Subsequently, Kuhn's observations on imipramine (1958) in the treatment of depression, and Schou's popularization of lithium (1968) for the treatment of mania widened the therapeutic scope of psychopharmacology.

On the other side of the coin from socially approved medical prescription of drugs was the widespread self-administration of drugs for recreation, pleasure, or self-medication. To be sure, for centuries or even millenia a small number of vegetable products had been used by large populations for their mental effects.

Alcohol as the primary ingredient in mead, wine, beer, and whiskey is probably the first and the most commonly consumed psychoactive drug, but it is closely challenged by caffeine (found in coffee, tea, and maté) and by nicotine (found in tobacco). Morphine and heroin (derived from opium), the tetrahydrocannabinols (found in hemp), and cocaine (from coca leaves) have also been used by smaller but still large numbers of people in order to achieve certain mental effects. An even greater number of botanical products have been used by a much smaller number of people.

However, the discovery of the peculiar mental actions of lysergic acid diethylamide (LSD) by Hofmann in 1943 spurred a tremendous scientific as well as underground interest in hallucinogenic or psychotogenic drugs (see Hofmann, 1959). Drug experimentation mostly by young adventurers became very popular. It probably reached a peak in the 1960s and may have abated somewhat since then. Another class of drugs discovered by Alles in the 1930s—the amphetamines —entered the popular arena of illicit drugs in the 1960s especially in the "hippie" drug culture (see Alles, 1959). Interest in a variety of hallucinogenic drugs, particularly LSD and mescaline, was stimulated in the same counterculture, first by Huxley (1954) and later by Leary (1968).

The social and legal problems spawned by these drugs remain with us still. In the mid-1970s drug experimentation with newer drugs seems to have waned somewhat, largely because of fears of toxic actions. Nevertheless, among the illicit drugs, opiates, marijuana, and hashish, use remains very high, and debate about the possible legalization or modification of penalties for trafficking or use of these continues.

The implications of psychoactive drug use, legal and illegal, therapeutic and recreational, are of course tremendous. Such drugs as marijuana and alcohol are obvious social facilitators. Despite numerous investigations, however, it is still not clear exactly what they do to behavior nor how they do it. The sociopharmacologist seeks to understand all the links in the chain of reaction of a particular drug from pharmacological aspects to the study of social structures, and the interactions of these. Some of the questions he poses are, what factors (usually social) prompted the initial use of a drug? What actions does the drug have on individual and social behavior? Does the individual's behavior differ, depending upon whether he is in a group or alone? What are the variables in the environment that influence the drug's action? What physiological mechanisms inside the individual are responsible for the drug's action? What factors contribute to repeated use of the drug? Are these social or pharmacological? Does repeated use change reaction to the drug? Is the tolerance or sensitization frequently described for many drugs in purely pharmacological terms in part, at least, due to change also

produce bizarre mental changes. However, one extremely popular drug, the effects of which are most certainly mediated through its cholinergic actions, is the alkaloid nicotine. It can produce profound effects on brain physiology (Domino, 1965) and also on behavior (Dunn, 1973). In many ways, the study of nicotine use is an instructive, valid, and relatively simple model for that of other drugs also leading to dependence.

Tobacco appears to be the only source of nicotine. The evidence that smoking is really nicotine-seeking behavior is only circumstantial (Jarvik, 1970*b*), but some animal studies indicate that this drug may be self-administered by monkeys (Deneau & Inoki, 1967). In humans the induction of smoking is clearly socially mediated, most frequently by peer pressure in early adolescence. Once smoking becomes established some tolerance and physiological dependence can develop, particularly in heavy smokers (Knapp, Bliss, & Wells, 1963). Before the report of the Surgeon-General (Health, Education, and Welfare, 1964) in the United States or those of the Royal College of Physicians in the United Kingdom almost all smokers carried on with the habit until their deaths.

In recent years various social pressures have been applied to discourage smoking, but it is a very difficult habit to break. Dependence upon heroin and other opioids is maintained in part by efforts of the subject to prevent the physical symptoms of withdrawal (according to Wikler, 1968). Smokers experience few if any physiological withdrawal symptoms and signs yet have a craving, frequently very intense, that can become so distracting as to interfere with activity. Administration of very small, controlled amounts of nicotine to heavy smokers can diminish smoking to some extent (Lucchesi, Schuster, & Emley, 1967).

On the other hand, some promising leads are provided by certain major tranquilizers, the antipsychotic phenothiazines or butyrophenones. It is now thought that the primary effect of these is to block in some way the actions of the important catecholamine, dopamine. It is theorized that there is dopamine excess or hypersensitivity in psychotic states such as schizophrenia and that this is reduced or blocked by the antipsychotic drug. Patients with parkinsonism are now known to be deficient in dopamine (Hornykiewicz, 1966). Thus, some well-known major unwanted effects of the antipsychotic drugs, parkinsonian or related extrapyramidal syndromes, provide an additional pointer to the role of dopamine as transmitter. Some rather effective antipsychotics, such as thioridazine, have a lesser tendency to produce extrapyramidal actions, perhaps because they also possess antiparkinson effects by virtue of their antimuscarinic anticholinergic effects. The rauwolfia alkaloids, such as reserpine, while effective antipsychotic drugs, also tend to produce psychiatric depression presumably by depleting stores of dopamine (among other substances they release).

There has also been speculation that aspects of what is called mood are controlled by another catecholamine, norepinephrine (Schildkraut, 1970). If production or utilization of norepinephrine is high in states of mania or well-being, and low in depression, drugs that may "stimulate" or improve mood such as amphetamine, or such antidepressant drugs as the tricyclics (imipramine or amitriptyline) or the monoamine oxidase inhibitor, tranylcypromine do so by copying the actions of norepinephrine, by stimulating the production or by inhibiting the destruction of norepinephrine at or near its site of action. Direct evidence for this theory is difficult to come by, first because objective measurement of mood is not easy and, second, because it is impossible to measure the concentration of norepinephrine directly in the brains of living human patients. Metabolites of norepinephrine in the urine have been estimated instead and this has given some suggestive results, but contamination by the huge peripheral output of norepinephrine from the sympathetic nervous system and adrenal medulla makes conclusions very difficult. The discovery in the urine (Maas, Fawcett, & Dekirmenjian, 1968) of a norepinephrine metabolite produced only by the brain promises to throw much light on the place of the catecholamines in affective disorders. Some investigators believe that lithium is useful in the treatment of mania because it facilitates the reuptake of norepinephrine. However, it also depresses the electrical excitability of the neuronal membrane. Amphetamine produces its actions either through mimicking the actions of dopamine and norepinephrine at the receptor site or by increasing the amount of catecholamine at the receptor. The tricyclic antidepressant drugs also increase the net amount of norepinephrine at the receptor by inhibiting the reuptake of catecholamines at the presynaptic site. Monoamine oxidase inhibitors prevent the metabolic degradation of catecholamines and thereby increase their concentration at the receptor. Although the evidence for the role of catecholamines in mood and mental disease is indirect, it is so consistent that it would be surprising if some totally different transmitter pathway were involved in the action of drugs used to regulate mood and ameliorate the psychoses.

The place of 5HT is still something of a mystery. It used to be thought that the actions of reserpine were due to its ability to release 5HT from storage, but it now appears that with some exceptions this was coincidence: catecholamine release is the important action. However, the hypothermic effects of reserpine are due to 5HT depletion, as is the reserpine-induced decrease in slow-wave sleep time, but the significance of these observations is unclear. The functional role of 5HT, if any, is unknown.

Whether the other putative transmitters mentioned above mediate drug action and, if so, how, is still less certain. It is certain that GABA, glycine, and glutamic acid have something to do with levels of excitability; they may also be involved in the actions of antiepileptic drugs and also analeptic drugs such as strychnine, picrotoxin, and pentylenetetrazol (Metrazol). Caffeine is thought to stimulate the action of cyclic AMP by inhibiting the enzyme, phosphodiesterase, that destroys it.

An increasing knowledge of the nature of neurotransmission will make possible a more rational approach to drug and behavioral therapy. One objective, clearly, is to be able to synthesize a drug, or series of drugs, that will have quite specific effects. We are still far from this. There are too many poorly understood links in the chain of events connecting stimulus and response. We are beginning to gain a primitive understanding of the biochemical and physiological processes underlying activation and sleep, or of the relationship between mood and emotion, but all the steps in the production of the behavioral responses characteristic of anger or fear are not yet spelled out. The darkness is even blacker when it comes to understanding perception, cognition, learning, and memory. These functions can be disrupted fairly easily but unselectively by hallucinogenic drugs, for example. They may also be facilitated under special circumstances (McGaugh, 1968) that are far from well defined as yet. Obviously, it is necessary to continue to approach the problem from both ends, the neurochemical and the behavioral, and to bear in mind that the behavioral evidence is profoundly affected by the social setting in which it is gathered—a fact that is only now coming to be appreciated.

## DRUGS AND SOCIAL BEHAVIOR

The effects of drugs upon social behavior and the effect of social variables upon drug effects can be looked at in many ways. From one point of view, a drug may first be considered as an independent variable influencing (1) the internal environment of an individual, then (2) his interactions with the external environment including the perception of stationary and moving objects, then (3) his perception of the social environment, which in its simplest form comprises one other individual, and finally, (4) his interactions with others, including friends, strangers, business associates, family, and political groupings. Interaction at each of these levels could be affected by a drug taken by the individual, and might be the focus of interest. Conversely, the behavior of the subject under study can be affected by a drug taken by any of those with whom he is in contact (Nowlis & Nowlis, 1956; Starkweather, 1959; Joyce, 1965).

The nature of the interaction itself is another factor, ranging from simple approach or withdrawal, up to complex verbal or written intellectual interactions. Any activity can be modulated, and measured, in terms of its speed, steadiness, accuracy, as well as the feeling tone accompanying it (e.g., aggressive or friendly).

The nature and interpretation of the evidence from neuropharmacology, or traditional psychopharmacology, also depend upon the drug-dependent variable chosen for measurement. Different drugs affect different systems; for example, one system that is sensitive to drugs is the activation system. Its state can be described by measures of sleep-wakefulness, electroencephalographic activity, and general motor activity. Most psychoactive drugs can be (and often are) crudely classified as depressants or stimulants of this and other systems, but these labels are unsatisfactory because the behavior (whether of an individual cell, an organ system, or a whole individual) frequently depends upon the contemporary state, as well as upon the dose used, and because depression of neural activity of a certain kind can in fact lead to stimulation at the overall behavioral level.

The remainder of this section is divided into three subsections, as follows:

1. Variables of primarily *internal* origin that modify drug action, such as personality differences and hereditary influences. In a neonate all factors susceptible to influence by drugs must be considered innate unless they have been acquired in intrauterine life (e.g., addiction to heroin). By later life, interaction with the environment will have produced fairly stable personality patterns, as well as acquired biochemical sensitivities, that are internalized and carried by the individual from place to place. Genetic influences, however, will persist throughout life and may be responsible for idiosyncratic drug reactions even in old age. There are also racial differences in drug sensitivity; some may be culturally determined, but some are certainly genetic (e.g., primaquine sensitivity among certain Mediterranean peoples, responses of American Indians or some oriental races to alcohol). Some variables of internal origin may last only for a very short time, although superimposed upon older and longer-lasting personality traits. Such variables as suggestibility, tolerance, and sensitization are subsumed in this section. Differences among personalities are still undefined, except theoretically in biochemical terms, but do induce variability in drug effects. Experimenter-induced and subject-induced expectation, placebo effects, and individual variations in drug responsiveness are also included in this section, although it is often difficult to decide whether such variables are external or internal to the organism.

2. Variables of primarily *external* origin deriving from the physical and social environment that modify drug action, such as anoxia at high altitude, temperature extremes, nutritional deficiencies, and stress. Since the type of task selected by the experimenter or used by the psychiatrist as a clinical measure is derived from the social environment, task effects are discussed in this section.

3. A comparison of drug responses in individual and group settings. After a

discussion of the variables influencing drug effects in the individual pharmacological experiments in group settings are considered. The final section also briefly considers certain social variables in recreational drug use: taking drugs for religious, artistic, and hedonistic purposes; the generally increasing tendency towards self-medication; and the problems of control of various forms of psychic deviance with psychoactive drugs.

## Variables of Internal Origin

### Genetic Factors

The proportionate roles of genetic and environmental factors in alcoholism have been subjected to extensive research, as exemplified by a study of the metabolism of ethanol (Vesell, Page, & Passananti, 1971). The rate of metabolism of ethanol as such has not been established as the physiological basis of alcoholism but as an undoubtedly important factor. When the rate of metabolism of a single dose (1 ml/kg) of 95% ethanol was compared in 14 sets of healthy twins, identical twins had smaller intrapair differences than fraternal twins, suggesting that genetic control was much greater than environmental. Other types of research with humans (studies of alcoholism in families, in adopted children, and in half sibs), as well as animal studies showing strain differences in sensitivity to and preference for alcohol, emphasize the importance of genetic factors (McClearn, 1973).

Another factor presumably having at least a partially inherited basis for differential drug effects on behavior is gender. Psychoactive drugs have been reported to affect males differently from females. Jaattela, Mannisto, Paatero, & Tuomisto (1971) studied the effects of diazepam (an antianxiety agent), diphenhydramine (an antihistamine) and placebo on mood, the Digit Symbol Substitution Test (DSST), and digit span in 270 healthy students, standardizing dosage for body weight. Diazepam decreased activity and impaired performance on the DSST and digit span in both males and females, but had very different sex-related mood effects; it decreased sociability, and caused withdrawal and increased depression in females, but it increased euphoria in men. Diphenhydramine, similarly, decreased activity and somewhat depressed performance on the mental tests in both sexes, and produced some euphoria in men, but not in women. This study, while demonstrating interesting gender differences in drug reactivity, is as little able to tell us what is genetically and what is culturally determined as are most studies of this kind. More light could possibly be thrown on this phenomenon if it were studied in individuals phenotypically and genotypically of opposite sexes, such as patients who have undergone sex change procedures or others with gender identity problems (Stoller, 1968), but such experimental designs are clearly open to other kinds of objection.

## Expectation

Drugs, whether endogenous or exogenous, do not trigger specific emotional states, but rather a more general pattern of physiological response which is interpreted by a person in the framework of his surroundings, and of those cognitions available to him (see Lennard, Epstein, Bernstein and Ransom, 1971). Thus, aspects of the social environment directly influence the type of reaction one may have to a drug. Schachter (1964) demonstrated that the response to injected epinephrine varied according to the expectation, or set, induced by the experimenter. Thus a racing heart induced by epinephrine can be associated with running up a staircase, a great fright, or sexual anticipation. Meaningfulness is imparted by the social cues and not by the drug alone.

Frankenhaeuser, Post, Hagdahl, and Wrangsjoe (1964) administered 200 mg of the sedative-hypnotic pentobarbital or placebo orally to 15 normal female students on a simple reaction-time task, identifying the pentobarbital to the subjects as either a "depressant" or an agent of "unknown effect," and the placebo always as a "depressant." Pulse rate, objective reaction time, subjective estimates of reaction time, and feelings of wakefulness decreased with all treatments, although not uniformly. When pentobarbital was introduced as a depressant, it produced the greatest impairment of reaction time, but when given the "unknown" label its effects did not differ from the placebo introduced as a depressant. Subjectively, in fact, the placebo produced a slightly greater effect in estimates of fatigue, sleepiness, inefficiency, and relaxation than did unlabeled pentobarbital, although the effect was nonsignificant. Since 200 mg is double the most commonly used hypnotic dose, these results are quite striking. This study (and also a similar one by Ross, Krugman, Lyerly, & Clyde, 1962) illustrates the importance of social setting. Almost any *individual* receiving 200 mg of pentobarbital in a quiet darkened room would go to sleep. There are limits, however, beyond which suggestibility cannot counteract the effects of a drug. Intravenous barbiturates will inevitably produce anesthesia no matter what the subject has been told, but the threshold varies considerably as a function of mental state.

Jones (1971) used 100 experienced marijuana smokers as subjects in a randomized double-blind experiment in which each was given either a marijuana cigarette containing 1 g of purified plant material and 9 mg of THC, or 1 g of plant material alone (placebo). Global ratings of intoxication were made 30 minutes after smoking and at the end of the 3-hour session during which subjects filled out the comprehensive 272-item Subjective Drug Effects Questionnaire (SDEQ).

The physiological effects of smoking marijuana were significant for all subjects (increase in pulse rate, decrease in salivation, increase in conjunctival injection) as estimated by differences between before and after scores, while no significant changes occurred after placebo. However, the drug affected frequent users (those who smoked more than seven cigarettes per week) more than infrequent users (those who smoked less than two per month), and in some cases the two groups differed significantly. Infrequent users significantly differentiated between the placebo and the active cigarette on the global intoxication scale, while frequent users did not, suggesting that the subjective set produced by smoking a familiar substance may be quite strong.

Evidently the rating of one's internal state depends on expectation, experience, and so on, as well as on specific physical responses. When Jones tested a smaller group of subjects (16), both individually and in groups, the effect of setting was vividly demonstrated. When tested as individuals, subjects were relaxed and drowsy (sedated), whereas when tested in a group, typical subjective responses were euphoria, elation, lack of sedation, and more reports of physical symptoms. Global ratings of intoxication were also higher. Thus, the effects of cognitive expectations, drug-use experience, and individual versus group setting were shown to be significant factors in the response.

This experiment illuminates the results of many psychoactive drug experiments. The subjects frequently have a rather good idea of what they are supposed to experience; if they are sophisticated and if informed consent has been required, the subjects tend to give the expected answers unless elaborate measures are taken to control for this.

*Personality*

Millions of words and thousands of papers have been written on ways of measuring psychological variables that determine drug effects or can be affected by drugs. Among the multitudes of measures some have become favorites. Thus "personality" is frequently measured by the Minnesota Multiphasic Test and "anxiety" by its derivative, the Taylor Manifest Anxiety Scale. Certain other mood scales are widely used including those for depression developed by Hamilton and by Zung. The varieties of perception and intellectual performance are so great that no one set of tests can be said to exhaustively describe all the variables. In addition to objective testing, which is difficult, the relatively easier procedure of subjective ratings, or the still easier procedure of uncontrolled anecdotal reporting, is common in psychopharmacological investigation.

Gottschalk, Gleser, Stone, and Kunkel (1969) developed the technique of content analysis of a 3-, 5-, or 10-minute monologue, speech, or written dream description sample. Scales for anxiety, hostility, social alienation–personality disorganization (schizophrenia) have been validated in order to assess various personality factors. The Gottschalk-Gleser hostility scale has been used to compare differences in outward and inward directed hostility in normals and patients with various pathological conditions, such as coronary artery disease and essential hypertension (Gottschalk, 1969). In a series of experiments using different classes of psychoactive drugs the technique successfully differentiated active ingredient and placebo on the various scales (Gottschalk et al., 1969). The hostility scale has also been used in psychopharmacological studies to measure changes in hostility level during treatment: hostility scores were reduced by perphenazine and chlordiazepoxide (tranquilizers), and increased following the antidepressant imipramine (Gottschalk, 1969).

Gottschalk accurately points out that different measurement techniques often yield different results. Adjective checklists are, by nature, obvious in their specification of symptomatology, and a more "natural" type of response from the subject may provide more reliable clues to his reactions. Whether this particular tool will be of general utility remains to be seen, but the development of subtle measures of drug effects as well as of personality factors is needed in sociopharmacology and should be actively encouraged.

### Placebo Response

A further consideration is the influence of personality in producing placebo reactions and variations in drug responsiveness. The aim is to identify those who react most strongly to suggestive descriptions of therapeutic effects.

Placebo effects have been widely studied and efforts made to sort out "reactor" personality types (Wolf, Doering, Clark & Hagans, 1957; Joyce, 1961). However, as various authors point out (Downing & Rickels, 1970; Evans, 1968), it may not even be possible to classify someone as a placebo reactor without delineating the circumstances, since the effects of cognition and of the specific situation influence the degree of placebo response. Indeed, the very existence of placebo reaction has been questioned, on the ground that those experimenters who expect to find placebo effects tend to find them (e.g., Joyce) whereas those who do not expect placebo effects, do not find them (e.g., Wolf et al.; Joyce, personal communication). Task-specific variables are undoubtedly also involved; Frankenhaeuser, Post, Hagdahl, and Wrangsjoe (1964) noted that placebo effects began to wear off after 80 minutes in a simple reaction-time task, and Lehmann and Knight (1960) found that speed was more affected by placebo than were measures of accuracy. Perhaps this means that activation levels are more subject to suggestion than are cognitive abilities. Placebo responses tend to decrease the number of trials or sessions, an effect ascribed to behavioral tolerance (Davis, Evans, & Gillis, 1969); pharmaceutical testing of new drugs or drug combinations has made use of this finding for some time (Porsolt, Joyce, & Summerfield, 1970).

If many post hoc attempts to describe placebo responders have not been very successful, neither have all the more ambitious predictions of placebo response in subjects identified as reactors before the experiment. For example, Freund, Krupp, Goodenough, and Preston (1972) studied the effects of $d$-amphetamine and placebo for 4 weeks on 64 obese female outpatients. Using the Oltman Portable Rod and Frame test for field dependence, subjects were classified as either "field dependent" and hence expected to be placebo reactors, whom the authors describe as relating well to the environment and external authority, or "field independent" placebo nonreactors who relied mainly on internal cues, depending less on external stimulation. The treatment was described to the patient as either a new or a known anorexiant, and half of each patient group was given each condition. Patients who received an active drug lost more weight than placebo patients during the entire study, showing that the active drug was effective. Patients in the "known drug" condition lost more weight than in the corresponding "new drug" condition. However, this result, for the first week of therapy, was not true for the 4-week total, demonstrating that such effects can be short-lived, and also that almost any kind of therapy for strong habits (e.g., smoking, drinking, eating, drug taking) is bound to have a brief period of success followed by relapse (Hunt & Matarrazo, 1973). The field-dependence classification did not seem to be especially useful, as the field-dependent patients lost no more weight than field-independent patients under the "known drug" condition. Either the choice of this classification was irrelevant to the prediction of placebo response, or the Oltman test did not separate the alleged types sufficiently.

A technically more sophisticated study of placebo response was made by Downing and Rickels (1970), who examined data on 388 neurotic outpatients from both clinics and private practice given placebos in several different experiments evaluating minor tranquilizers or antidepressants. The three measures of placebo response selected were changes in the severity of emotional and somatic symptomatology, and the amount of overall improvement as rated by both doctor and patient. Demographic information, the clinical history and the nature of the present complaint, and doctor-patient relationship were used to predict placebo response in a multiple-regression analysis.

The full set of 73 variables accounted for only 28% of the variance in placebo response; a stepwise search procedure produced a reduced set of variables that accounted for 19% of the variance. Lower social class and associated conditions (less formal education, unstable marital relationship, and lack of insight into emotional illness), a brief term of illness with a favorable prognosis, and lower initial level of depression predicted three separate measures of placebo response. The remarkably small proportion of variance attributable to identified variables by such a powerful form of data analysis may seem disappointing, but still the fact implies that prediction of placebo reaction is possible. Joyce (1961) was able to make better-than-chance predictions of placebo response from various psychological measures, but the best predictor was placebo reaction on a previous occasion.

Variability in drug responsiveness is probably closely related to placebo reactivity. DiMascio (1969) discussed three experiments on normal subjects in which there were no overall differences between response to drugs (chlorpromazine, imipramine, various minor tranquilizers) and placebo. Reanalyzing the data after dividing the subjects into personality types A and B (based on a previous analysis of differential drug reactivity), he found separate responses to the drugs, although not to placebo; for example (and perhaps not surprisingly) imipramine reduced depression and anxiety only in subjects initially high on either of these symptoms. Therefore, "normals" only respond to such drugs if there is a chance for the drugs to show clinical relevance. DiMascio nevertheless argues for the use of normal subjects in testing clinical agents given proper selection, since post hoc analyses remain exactly that. Only the successful prediction of clinical results using preselected groups will validate the division of subjects by personality type.

However, a similar approach using preselected and appropriate patients would appear to be more useful. For example, Slater and Kastenbaum (1966) found personality differences between geriatric patients who reacted to thioridazine or d-amphetamine in a clinically favorable direction and those who reacted in the opposite direction.

There are not only differences between patients or subjects, but differences of state from moment to moment or from episode to episode. These too will modify drug response in different ways. For instance, Riklan (1972) analyzed the behavioral alterations that occur when L-dopa is administered to geriatric parkinsonian patients, such as the alleviation or induction of depression, or changes leading either to disorientation and paranoid ideation or alertness and improved cognitive functioning. He hypothesized a general increase in activation, which, depending on the patient's state, would lead to directional changes in various functions.

### Paradoxical Effects

The most prominent example of so-called "paradoxical" drug effects is provided by the effects of central nervous system stimulants on already "hyperactive" children. Some critics of this treatment claim that drugs are used to control, or tranquilize, children who are otherwise difficult to discipline. Whatever the motives of those who use drugs for this purpose (the frequency with which this nonmedical diagnosis is accepted by prescribing physicians is probably unique in psychiatry), the paradoxical effect is the behavioral deactivation produced by a stimulant. Conners has comprehensively described this kind of hyperactivity and evaluation of the effects of stimulants, particularly $d$-amphetamine and methylphenidate (Conners, 1971a, 1971b; Conners, Kramer, Rothschild, Schwartz, & Stone, 1971; Conners, 1973). He points out that there is really no paradox. The total amount of activity remains the same or even increases, but the *quality* changes, becoming more directed and less diffuse. The heterogeneity of the patient sample makes it very difficult to evaluate the effects, whether these are of no change or intellectual and behavioral improvement. Subgroups from the overall population obtained by cluster analysis of individual behavior profiles respond differentially to the drugs; differences in such physiological measures as cortical evoked potential to visual and auditory stimuli are also obtained.

The psychological function most affected by the stimulant drugs appears to be attention, but even here the change is dependent upon a particular behavior constellation. Children who showed significant improvement on Harris-Goodenough Figure Drawings, which yield an IQ score representing the child's ability to reproduce the human figure, had a low verbal IQ, a relatively good performance IQ, and did not present behavior problems at home (Conners, 1971a). The improvement was attributed to better ability to pay attention to directions, selectively attend to the task, and to persevere at it. Recently, Conners (1973) has factor and cluster analyzed a large battery of tests administered to children with minimal brain dysfunction. He examined the neurological and physiological differences among six homogeneous groups, one of which resembled the normal. The groups differed in motor development, averaged evoked response between the two hemispheres, and response to medication. This type of analysis should improve the choice of treatment for children with minimal brain dysfunction and other behavioral disturbances. The use of stimulants in appropriate cases to improve attention and social behavior is clearly valuable and an important area for research in sociopharmacology, since communication and other social skills are apparently improved by the use of stimulants for such children.

## Variables of External Origin

Physical as well as social factors in the environment are relevant to sociopharmacology. These can produce biochemical changes within an organism, altering its physiological and psychological functioning, and the effects of a drug upon resultant behavior. Physical factors include hypoxia experienced at high altitudes, extremes of temperature, isolation, and even differences in the strength of the gravitational field. Social factors include various types of stress and the nature of the task used in an experiment.

The distinction between internal and external factors is often difficult, however, inasmuch as all external factors ultimately manifest their actions by some effect on the brain (internal) and thereby on behavior. Neither is it always easy to disinguish the social from the physical—nutritional deficiency for example, especially in infancy, has elements of both. But the distinction is convenient, if not precise, and is used in this section.

*Altitude*

Decrements in physical and intellectual performance occur at high altitudes, but stimulants counteract performance deficits induced by hypoxia (Evans, 1970). And although most studies are conducted in simulations of high altitude, reports by mountain climbers corroborate the experimental observations, including the use of stimulants to alleviate the suffering (for example see Hornbein, 1968).

The interaction of drugs and acute hypoxia on mice and rats in a hypobaric chamber has been studied (DeFeo, Baumel, & Lal, 1970). The duration of sleep induced by pentobarbital or chloral hydrate was increased fivefold, and by barbital twentyfold, for mice (but rats were far less sensitive). Hypoxic mice also slept and remained asleep at doses of barbiturates that would have been inadequate to induce sleep at normal oxygen concentrations. Hypoxia caused a much greater reduction of temperature in mice (5.8 °C) than in rats (2.5 °C). The lowered temperature due to hypoxia greatly lengthened the sleeping time under barbital. The authors suggested that central nervous system depression was enhanced by the experimental conditions, and supported this by demonstrating a lower threshold to convulsants.

A low oxygen level has a remarkably long-lasting effect in people, even those acclimatized to life at high altitudes, such as Indians of the high Andes or the Sherpa tribesmen of the Himalayas. It is frequently necessary for them to descend to lower altitudes to cope with such events as childbirth or illness.

*Temperature*

Though unable to adapt to more than relatively slight changes in the oxygen content of the air, man is insulated physiologically to withstand quite a wide range of temperature differences, and appropriate clothing helps even further. The effects of temperature on drug actions in animal and man are presented in an

brain weight, increased brain monoamine concentrations, and decreased activity of the liver enzymes synthesizing 5HT were found in the animals fed diets low in protein, but the behavioral and physiological abnormalities were "normalized" by the administration of pyrithioxin (Encephabol, a neurotropic agent supposedly reducing the permeability of the blood brain barrier to phosphates) between days 48–58. Early malnutrition did not adversely affect the learning or retention of an active avoidance habit or visual discrimination, but the abnormal manner of responding employed by the adult rat was prevented by pyrithioxin administration.

Failure to find changes in behavioral (individual and social) responses arising from early starvation may be due to the employment of inadequately sensitive methods of observation. The area remains of obvious interest to sociopharmacologists, however.

## Stress

Conditions of stress or severe extremes of homeostatic mechanisms (of which malnutrition may be considered a special long-term example) alter the physiological state of the organism, affecting hormonal balances and central nervous system functioning. Thus it follows that drug responses should also be altered by stress.

Social interactions such as crowding, aggression, fighting, or fleeing are often the cause of stress in members of the group. That is, stimulus conditions perceived as uncomfortable or dangerous can result in individual homeostatic changes. Stress may cause profound central and peripheral changes which are not always adaptive. Hypoxia, hypothermia, exercise, and psychological stress all cause activation of the sympathetic nervous system and bring about "stress hypoglycemia," in which glucose metabolism is changed and insulin secretion inhibited by epinephrine. Since the CNS itself is not sensitive to insulin, it utilizes the available glucose. So these changes in insulin regulation and glucose metabolism underlie certain altered responses to drugs during stress (Porte and Robertson, 1973).

Alcoholism is an excellent example of a drug-utilizing response to social pressures. The effect of psychological stress upon the drinking behavior, mood, and psychopathology of chronic alcoholics was studied over a 32-day period by Allman, Taylor, and Nathan (1972). Subjects "earned" their alcohol by responding in an operant conditioning paradigm. They were stressed by being led to believe that they were not working hard enough to receive alcohol. Most alcohol was consumed when periods of stress coincided with opportunities for group contact, and least when stress was accompanied by isolation.

## Task Conditions

The judgment of whether or not a drug is having an effect often rests upon the nature of the task. General guidelines for drug sensitivity and drug resistance of tasks have been proposed (Evans, 1970). The decision between alternative measures is partly a social judgment, but neither this nor the much less trivial influence of the extent of the experimenter's participation in the experimental situation have yet received systematic, or indeed any adequate theoretical or practical consideration. Leaving these important matters on one side, for the moment, it is still necessary to review the factors inherent in the task that may *directly* influence performance. Measures of aspects of performance that can fluctuate, such as descriptions of mood, tend to be drug sensitive, whereas those measuring relatively stable aspects such as IQ or personality factors (Joyce, 1971) tend to be drug resistant. Numerous other aspects of the task affect performance as influenced by drugs. Tests of speed are more sensitive than tests of accuracy. A task in which feedback is delayed is more sensitive to drugs than one in which feedback is immediate. Complex tasks may be more sensitive than simple ones. These general principles are less and less reliable as the number of factors increases.

Performance on psychomotor tasks, and those involving attention and perception, is generally facilitated by stimulants and depressed by barbiturates, but there is still disagreement over whether the effect is a direct enhancement of attention or a reduction in fatigue (Herrington, 1967; Talland & Quarton, 1965, 1966; Weiss & Laties, 1962). There seems to be no general facilitation of intellectual performance by stimulants (Weiss & Laties, 1962), but the effects can be modified by experience with the task, or with the drug, or both. Thus Davis, Evans, and Gillis (1969) reported very complex effects of amphetamine and chlorpromazine on multiple cue probability learning (MCPL) tasks. These drugs impaired learning of simple MCPL problems and had no effect upon complex ones, yet if the subject was experienced in the task the effect of drugs was decreased. Task difficulty and behavioral experience complicate the interpretation of drug effects upon intellectual functions. Experience with the drug itself might also be expected to diminish the influence of the drug on performance, an important point for people given psychoactive drugs to bear in mind when—despite the injunctions of their doctor or the manufacturer—they need to drive cars or operate other machinery.

The relationship of drug sensitivity to task difficulty has not been systematically studied. Experimenters have used a variety of drugs and doses, different subject populations, and cognitive tasks that cannot be easily ordered on a scale of difficulty. Evans (1968, 1970) maintained that tests of complex functioning were more sensitive to drugs than those of simple functioning, yet, in the work mentioned above, Davis et al. (1969) found the opposite effect. Their task was quite different from those most frequently used in psychology experiments that measure learning and memory of meaningful or nonmeaningful materials. There are certainly reasons for the different conclusions reached in perfectly valid experiments, but they are far from clear.

Latz (1968) summarized a number of studies on cognitive test performance using a variety of psychoactive agents (major and minor tranquilizers, and antidepressants). He concluded that performance on cognitively complex tasks is *not* differentially more drug sensitive and that decrements in complex performance largely result from disturbance of subsidiary functions. He arranged tasks in increasing order of difficulty, but without defining his criteria of complexity, as follows: cancellation tests and symbol-copying tests, coding tests, arithmetic tests, memory for digits, learning of nonsense syllables and paired associates. It appears that the influence of speed of performance was not taken into account. It is also unsatisfactory to compare tasks involving motor coordination with cognitive learning in terms of task difficulty. One would expect performance on these tests to be impaired by the drugs discussed in his review, which often cause motor slowing.

Centrally active drugs affect cognitive functions such as reasoning, learning, and memory as well as arousal, attention, perception, motivation, and mood. Since the separation of functions is difficult, the interactions among cognitive and noncognitive variables often remain confounded. For example, if the subject has not paid *attention* to the items in a learning task, he will show a decrement in performance which may be falsely attributed to a *learning* deficit. The experiment by Hill, Belleville, and Wikler (1957) discussed below illustrates the powerful effects of varying motivation on reaction-time performance while keeping drug dose constant. Cognitive functions have not been thoroughly studied under conditions of varying interest, motivation, or social influences.

Meaningfulness and interest value of materials is another task-relevant variable. Stimulants are more effective in boring situations. In a monotonous reaction-time task, Frankenhaeuser, Myrsten, Post, and Johansson (1971) found that cigarette smoking facilitated performance and prevented decrements from fatigue; however, this effect of smoking did not increase performance above the nonfatigued level. A second study (Myrsten, Andersson, Frankenhaeuser, & Mardh, 1972) substantiated these results using habitual smokers as subjects in a "tense and loaded" task, choice reaction time (RT). Cigarette smoking in the simple RT condition prevented the deterioration over time that occurred in the control condition, as before, and smoking during the choice RT task led to an actually significant improvement in performance. The stimulant effects of smoking had a simple facilitative effect on performance whether stressed or not. Myrsten, Post, Frankenhaeuser, and Johansson (1972) next divided cigarette smokers by means of a questionnaire into low-arousal versus high-arousal categories, depending on whether they smoked more in boring situations or in anxiety-inducing, exciting situations. A visual-vigilance task and a complex sensorimotor task respectively represented low- and high-arousal situations. Low-arousal subjects performed better and felt better only after smoking in the low-arousal situation, and high-arousal subjects were favorably affected by smoking only in the high-arousal situation. These experiments show that task-imposed stress and drug effects can even interact differently depending on motives for smoking. A physiological basis for high-arousal and low-arousal smoking has not been reported yet.

An important task-related variable that is seldom manipulated in humans is incentive. That drug effects on performance differ as incentive value (and thus presumably motivation) is varied was demonstrated in a fascinating experiment by Hill, Belleville, and Wikler (1957). Former morphine addicts serving federal sentences for narcotics violations were given, under blind conditions, either placebo, morphine sulfate 15 mg i.m., or pentobarbital sodium 250 mg i.m. 50 minutes before performing a simple visual-motor RT task. All subjects also received morphine sulfate for serving in the experiment in one of four incentive conditions: (1) Low Incentive—all subjects received the same dose, given 1 week before the experiment; (2) Standard 1 Incentive—all subjects received the same dose, given immediately after the trial (3) High Incentive—the size of the dose given after the trial depended on the subject's speed of response; and (4) Standard 2 Incentive—resembling Standard 1, but using subjects who had previously served in the High Incentive condition, and feedback. Social variables undoubtedly entered because subjects considered that the High Incentive condition represented a competitive situation.

Depending on the incentive condition, the effects of pentobarbital and morphine varied from *stimulant* to *depressant*, or had no *effect at all*. Had only one incentive condition been used, much information would have been lost and that which remained would probably have misled. Performance was changed most by the different kinds of incentive under pentobarbital; reaction times were slowest in the Low Incentive condition and fastest under High Incentive. The differences were remarkable. Pentobarbital seemed to enhance motivational variables, the changes due to incentives when subjects were treated with morphine being much smaller. Reaction time in the Low Incentive condition was not significantly different from Standard 1 Incentive; significantly faster reaction times occurred only under the two High Incentive conditions. In comparison with placebo, however, morphine acted as a "stimulant" (i.e., brought about a relatively faster reaction time) under Low Incentive conditions and as a "depressant" (i.e., slowed reaction time in comparison with placebo) under the Standard 2 or High Incentive conditions. Morphine thus seemed to lessen the influence of motivational variables. The authors concluded that motivation must be controlled in order to observe a specific drug effect, and that ". . . drugs exert 'specific' effects on particular motivations . . . differences in the attractiveness of drugs for different persons may be partly explained on the basis that motivations acceptable to the subject can be enhanced and unacceptable ones suppressed by the use of particular chemical agents [Hill et al., 1957, p. 35]."

## The Individual and the Group—Drugs and Social Behavior

Nonhuman species that manifest social behavior include ants, hive-building insects, and many species between these and the primates, all of which exhibit complex cooperative interactions and live in groups. All species, of course, exhibit some social behavior in relation to sex, and a majority in relation to rearing of the young, aggression, and other forms of communication as well. Some of these aspects of social behavior can be artificially induced in an individual setting with drugs, and their occurrence modified in a group setting. The experiments discussed in this section report drug-induced behavior changes in solitary and group settings that are related in some way to social activity.

Social behavior can be easily studied in both laboratory and natural settings. Research with animals has the advantage that potentially toxic and other powerful agents in doses that could not be given to humans can be employed. Generalization to human behavior must always be cautious, especially in the area of social interaction, where man's communicative ability is outstandingly different from that of infrahumans.

Some of the most physiologically "natural" agents that influence social behavior are sex hormones. Hormonal influences on sexual behavior have been thoroughly studied in animals (Beach & Merari, 1970). Injection of estrogen into female dogs increases sexual interest and activity in both males and females, and subsequent injection of the females with progesterone further increases the males' excitation and copulatory activity. It is interesting to note that the individual differences in the preferences of the males for the several female dogs were accentuated by the hormonal treatments. Sex hormones can also alter the relative position of individuals in dominance hierarchies (Lehrman, 1964; Beach & Merari, 1970; Whalen, 1966).

In humans the psychological and behavioral changes following treatment with oral contraceptives (which are usually a mixture of sex hormones: progestogens and estrogens) have been less carefully examined than one would expect, considering that these drugs are now routinely administered to millions of women throughout the world. In one of the few studies made, the effects of oral contraceptive agents were compared in women of child-bearing age for the first 2 months of administration, the time during which most mood changes as well as other disturbances are most frequently reported (Kane, Lipton, Krall, & Obrist, 1970). Mestranol alone (a progestogen) produced few biochemical or behavioral changes, but a combination of an estrogen and a progestogen produced mood changes, mild physical discomfort (nausea, fatigue, appetite change), and changes in catecholamine metabolism. Substances with effects similar to those that modify behavior in mice (Bruce & Parkes, 1961), or control breeding in insects (Comfort, 1971) have been postulated for men (or women) but not yet conclusively demonstrated. Drug effects on social behavior are much easier to study in animals than in humans because experiments can be designed and executed more easily. Though care must be exercised in making inferences from animal models, these are nevertheless relevant to human sociopharmacology. However, an animal model of human psychopathology (for example, schizophrenia) may be unsatisfactory even if the basic cause of the disorder in humans is not biochemical but socially determined, because the human social determinants cannot be satisfactorily represented in animals.

Van der Poel and Remmelts (1971) demonstrated a dose-response curve for the effects of scopolamine, an antimuscarinic anticholinergic drug with central and peripheral actions, on solitary and group behavior in rats. Drug effects on individual behavior were visible mainly in changes in maintenance behavior (grooming, washing, vibrating); there were no consistent changes in exploratory behavior. A dose-related change in social behavior was shown principally in decreases in aggressive, defensive (except crouch), and play elements of behavior. The behavior of untreated partner rats ran parallel to that of the treated partners; as the treated rat became less aggressive so did the untreated partner. Methylscopolamine, an agent with only peripheral actions, had no effect in the same dose range. This study showed that the behavior of even a nondrugged animal can be affected through the social reactions of a drugged partner, and in a dose-related manner.

Borgesova and Krsiak (1972) demonstrated that alcohol also decreases aggressive and defensive behavior of untreated partner rats. The solitary behavior of the treated animal was unchanged but its social behavior decreased. A similar effect had earlier been shown in mice (Borgesova, Kadlecova, & Krsiak, 1971). Untreated partners fled from treated mice and exhibited fewer aggressive responses. Interestingly, the partners of mice treated with chlordiazepoxide, a minor tranquilizer, became *more* aggressive, showing fewer defensive and escape reactions. Physical or visual contact was apparently needed for the untreated partner to be "nonworker" went to work. This social effect was dose-dependent and only occurred in pairs where the worker rat was treated. Chlorpromazine exerted a similar but smaller effect; the performance curves did not cross. Amobarbital produced ataxia and anesthesia. The authors attribute the inversion of the curve under $\Delta^9$-THC to perceptual changes leading to deconditioning of worker rats without loss of motivation.

Johnson (1972) has discussed how stimulus significance could be affected by different drugs. For example, social interaction might be reduced by chlorpromazine because the significance of sensory stimuli is reduced. Lithium decreases activity and blocks the orienting response to stimuli so that habituation is prevented; responsiveness to stimuli is therefore altered. Such an interpretation might be applied to the experiment of Masur, Martz, and Carlini (1972) discussed above.

The effects of several categories of psychoactive drugs (antidepressants, hypnotics, antipsychotics, MAOI's, analeptics, psychotomimetics, and minor tranquilizers) on the behavior of single and entire colonies of oriental hornets (Vespa orientalis F.), in the nest and in flight, resembled those in mammals, including man (Floru, Ishay, & Gitter, 1969).

Many animal studies showing profound changes in social behavior following the administration of psychoactive drugs are attempts to model human disease processes and explore their biochemical mechanisms; for example, the relation of deficiencies of dopamine and norepinephrine to human depressive disorders.

Redmond, Maas, Kling and Dekirmenjian (1971) administered alpha-methylparatyrosine (AMPT) for 6 and 13 weeks, respectively, to two Macaca speciosa monkeys of a social group of five. AMPT inhibits the synthesis of dopamine and norepinephrine by the enzyme tyrosine hydroxylase but does not affect other brain amines. The treated animals assumed a withdrawn posture and showed little motor activity; they initiated fewer social interactions such as grooming, threats, and attacks. However, the nontreated animals continued to interact with the treated ones, who remained responsive, so that the total number of social responses and social-sexual presentations did not decline. An attempt to reverse the AMPT-induced behavioral changes in one of the primates by giving L-dopa together with AMPT for 6 weeks was unsuccessful, perhaps because the dose of L-dopa may have been insufficient to return norepinephrine levels to normal; catecholamine excretion in the urine remained low. When treatment was discontinued, the behavior of both monkeys returned to normal.

Parachlorophenylalanine (PCPA) decreases the synthesis of 5HT, another monoamine possibly implicated in the depressive illnesses. Two animals in each of two groups of five monkeys were treated for 4 weeks with PCPA (Redmond,

Maas, Kling, Graham, & Dekirmenjian, 1971). These animals became quite ill but maintained their normal level of social activity and interest. The authors concluded that the catecholamines, but not the indolamines, are implicated in this form of experimental "depression" in this species.

In the most recent of this series of experiments (Redmond, Hinricks, Maas, & Kling, 1973), six wild adult macaque monkeys *(M. mulatta)* were captured from existing colonies on Guayacan Island, Puerto Rico. Two females and one male were each given a total of 30 mg of 6-hydroxydopamine in five intraventricular injections, an amount that in the laboratory is sufficient to deplete whole-brain norepinephrine by 69%; the remaining three macaques were sham operated. The drugged animals appeared healthier in the laboratory than those treated in the earlier experiments, but "unemotional." When all were returned to their natural environment 4 days later, the sham operated animals rejoined their social groups and behaved normally. The two treated females, however, did not return immediately to their social group and certain of their social behaviors were significantly decreased when they finally did return; they submitted to attack, showed less aggressive behavior, and became the lowest ranking of the adults observed. The treated male became solitary. There were subtle changes in physical characteristics, such as slumped posture, staring, and altered gait. The changes resembled those in caged *M. speciosa* given AMPT (Redmond, Maas, Kling, & Dekirmenjian, 1971). Thus the observations on natural behaviors, family situation, and social groups were extended and supported the hypothesis that the catecholamines are involved in complex behavior. The general implication of all these animal studies is that aggressiveness and other kinds of interactive behavior can be markedly influenced by drugs.

An interesting and highly controversial extrapolation from these studies was made in the inaugural address of Kenneth B. Clark (1971) as president of the American Psychological Association. He proposed that drugs shown to curb aggressiveness in animals (perhaps with some modification and improvement) might be used to curb the aggressive impulses of national leaders and promote cooperation instead of competition. This suggestion elicited many protests, and fears of *1984* and thought control were expressed. However, there is some merit to the somewhat oversimplified suggestion. The precipitous action of a mad leader can plunge nations into war. There are many historical examples.

Since the rise of hallucinogenic drugs to popularity and some notoriety several years ago, research on them has continued to increase dramatically. Siegel (1973*b*) reviewed the effects of hallucinogens on individual and group behavior in animals. Hypothermia, ataxia, and sedation are the primary physical effects of hallucinogens on solitary rodents. Such a "sick" state may have little effect on an

Experiments on animals using drugs for the treatment of mental illness (e.g., antipsychotics, antidepressants, tranquilizers, barbiturates) are often interesting but seldom illuminate the problem of human social pathology. The information may become more useful when more complex controlled experimental designs can be used.

The most valuable of the animal experiments at present are probably those on alterations in the social behavior of primates after brain catecholamine depletion, a possible basis for understanding some human depressive disorders.

The use of drugs in group process experiments with human subjects, the actual subject matter of human sociopharmacology, is just beginning. Some of the problems are typified by Schachter's observation that the *a priori* effect of an unidentified drug is nonspecific, and is interpreted in accordance with the subject's cognitive expectations (Schachter, 1964).

## Self-Medication

The widespread self-administration of drugs outside a medical context is referred to by such names as "drug abuse" or "recreational drug use." A more neutral term such as "self-medication" would include illicit use of illicit drugs such as heroin or marijuana, or licit use of others like alcohol or nicotine, as well as the large volume of over-the-counter, self-prescribed drugs. The social problems caused by the use of these and other drugs have been extensively discussed in recent years. For any drug in these categories one can ask at least four kinds of questions: (1) What effects does it have? (2) What harm (or what good) does it do? (3) Why do people use it? (4) How can you make them (or help them) to stop? The present book is chiefly concerned with the first question, but sociopharmacology is also clearly concerned with the other three questions as well.

With respect to the question of preventing drug abuse the following, among many possible examples, may be put forward. If a drug could be developed that would produce the same internal cues as the drug one desires to give up (e.g., nicotine), and (1) could be safely administered by a route other than the normal (e.g., smoking), and (2) would block the pharmacological effects (as do the narcotic antagonists), then it might be possible to help people to stop using a given drug. Pharmacological reinforcement contributing to the habit could be extinguished more easily than by the exercise of "will power" or other psychological exercises that are inadequate by themselves.

Answers to the questions posed depend on the one hand upon studies of motivation and on the other on evidence from epidemiology and toxicology, and have been treated at length, although seldom very well, by many authors. Group dynamics plays an extremely important role in the onset and cessation of drug habits but are difficult to manipulate in humans. Similar problems are involved in the making and breaking of nondrug habits to which the technology of psychotherapy is relevant. A sociopharmacologist could well be concerned with aspects of communication in these situations. Different approaches must be used with different groups as well as with different drugs, however. It is by no means certain that questionnaires would produce reliable information from middle-aged housewives who overuse barbiturates and amphetamines, or participant observation from a group of youths misusing opioids and hallucinogens. There are few, if any, studies that go to the methodological depth necessary to answer questions of this kind in work on self-medication.

A critical review of the work done in connection with self-medication, the work necessary and the techniques used or available, belongs to another kind of book than this one, with authors (and editors) of different competences if not necessarily different interests. Since the present book is, however, concerned with the experimental study of the social effects of drugs widely used in the treatment of mental illness, the methodology and results of psychological investigation in the clinic must be discussed. This is done in the following chapter.

## REFERENCES

Aghajanian, G. K. The effects of LSD on raphe nuclei neurons. In F. O. Schmitt, G. Adelman, T. Melnechuk and F. G. Worden (Eds.), *Neurosciences research symposium summaries*. Vol. 5. Cambridge, Mass.: MIT Press, 1971.

Alles, G. A. Some relations between chemical structure and physiological action of mescaline and related compounds. In H. A. Abramson (Ed.), *Fourth conference on neuropharmacology*. New York: Josiah Mac, Jr. Foundation, 1959.

Allman, L. R., Taylor, A., and Nathan, P. Group drinking during stress: Effects on drinking behavior, affect and psychopathology. *American Journal of Psychiatry*, 1972, **129,** 669–678.

Back, K. W., Oelfke, S. R., Brehm, M. L., Bogdonoff, M. D., and Nowlin, J. B. Physiological and situational factors in psychopharmacological experiments. *Psychophysiology*, 1970, **6,** 749–760.

Barron, F., Jarvik, M. E., and Bunnell, S., Jr. The hallucinogenic drugs. *Scientific American*, 1964, **210,** 3–11.

Beach, F. A. and Merari, A. Coital behavior in dogs: V. Effects of estrogen and progesterone on mating and other forms of social behavior in the bitch. *Journal of Comparative and Physiological Psychology*, 1970, **70,** 1–22.

Benesova, O., Frankova, S. Tikal, K., Benes, V., and Kunz, K. The effects of pyrithioxin (Encephabol Merck) on behavior, learning and biochemical variables of brain in rats malnourished in early life. I. Individual and social behavior of rats in relation to brain monoamines and liver tryptophan-pyrrolase activity. *Activitas Nervosa Superior*, 1972, **14,** 172–174.

Borgesova, M., Kadlecova, O., and Krsiak, M. Behavior of untreated mice to alcohol—or chlordiazepoxide-treated partners. *Activitas Nervosa Superior*, 1971, **13**, 206–207.

Borgesova, M. and Krsiak, M. Effect of alcohol on a diadic interaction in rats. *Activitas Nervosa Superior*, 1972, **14**, 169–170.

Brecher, E. M. *Licit and illicit drugs*. Boston: Little, Brown, 1972.

Bruce H. M. and Parkes, A. S. An olfactory block implantation in mice. *Journal of Reproduction and Fertility*, 1961, **2**, 195–196.

Burn, J. H. and Hobbs, R. A test for tranquilizing drugs. *Archives Internationales de Pharmacodynamie et de Thérapie*, 1958, **113**, 290–295.

Callear, J. F. F. and Van Gestel, J. F. E. An analysis of the results of field experiments in pigs in the UK and Ireland with the sedative neuroleptic azaperone. *The Veterinary Record*, 1971, **89**, 453–458.

Cheek, F. E. and Holstein, C. Lysergic acid diethylamide tartrate (LSD-25) dosage levels, group differences and social interaction. *Journal of Nervous and Mental Diseases*, 1971, **153**, 133–147.

Clark, K. B. The pathos of power: a psychological perspective. *American Psychologist*, 1971, **26**, 1047–1057.

Comfort, A. Likelihood of human pheromones. *Nature*, 1971, **230**, 432–433.

Conners, C. K. Recent drug studies with hyperkinetic children. *Journal of Learning Disabilities*, 1971, **4**, 14–19. *(a)*

Conners, C. K. The effect of stimulant drugs on human figure drawings in children with minimal brain dysfunction. *Psychopharmacologia*, 1971, **19**, 329–333. *(b)*

Conners, C. K. Psychological assessment of children with minimal brain dysfunction. *Annals, New York Academy of Sciences*, 1973, **205**, 283–302.

Conners, C. K., Kramer, R., Rothschild, G. H., Schwartz, L., and Stone, A. Treatment of young delinquent boys with diphenylhydantoin sodium and methylphenidate. *Archives of General Psychiatry*, 1971, **24**, 156–160.

Cooper, J. R., Bloom, F. E., and Roth, R. H. *The biochemical basis of neuropharmacology*. New York: Oxford University Press, 1970.

Davis, K. E., Evans, W. O., and Gillis, J. S. The effects of amphetamine and chlorpromazine on cognitive skills and feelings in normal adult males. In W. O. Evans and N. S. Kline (Eds.), *The psychopharmacology of the normal human*. Springfield: Charles C. Thomas, 1969.

De Feo, J. J., Baumel, I., and Lal, H. Drug environment interactions: acute hypoxia and chronic isolation. *Federation Proceedings*, 1970, **29**, 1985–1990.

Delay, J., Deniker, P., and Harl, J. M. Utilisation en therapeutique psychiatrique d'une phenothiazine d'action centrale elective (4560 RP). *Annales Medico-Psychologiques (Paris)*, 1952, **110**, 112–117.

Deneau, G. A. and Inoki, R. Nicotine self-administration in monkeys. *Annals of the New York Academy of Sciences*, 1967, **142**, 277–279.

Di Mascio, A. The use of "normals" in predicting clinical utility of psychotropic drugs. In W. O. Evans and N. S. Kline (Eds.), *The psychopharmacology of the normal human*. Springfield: Charles C. Thomas, 1969.

Dobbing, J. Undernutrition and the developing brain. In C. R. B. Joyce (Ed.), *Psychopharmacology, dimensions and perspectives*. London: Tavistock, 1968.

Domino, E. F. Some behavioral actions of nicotine. In U. S. von Euler (Ed.), *Tobacco alkaloids and related compounds*. Oxford: Pergamon, 1965.

Downing, R. W. and Rickels, K. The prediction of placebo response in anxious and depressed outpatients. In J. R. Wittenborn, S. C. Goldberg, and P. R. A. May (Eds.), *Psychopharmacology and the individual patient*. New York: Raven, 1970.

Dunn, W. L. *Smoking behavior: Motives and incentives*. Washington, D. C.: V. H. Winston, 1973.

Edwards, A. E. and Cohen, S. The attenuation of the external environment and the LSD effect. In W. O. Evans and N. S. Kline (Eds.), *The psychopharmacology of the normal human*. Springfield: Charles C. Thomas, 1969.

Eichenwald, H. F. and Fry, P. C. Nutrition and learning. *Science*, 1969, **163**, 644–648.

Evans, W. O. The psychopharmacology of the normal human: trends in research strategy. In D. H. Efron (Ed.), *Psychopharmacology, a review of progress 1957–1967*. (USPHS pub. No. 1836) Washington, D. C.: U. S. Government Printing Office, 1968.

Evans, W. O. Interaction of factors in the external environment upon the actions of psychotropic drugs in humans. *Federation Proceedings*, 1970, **29**, 1994–1999.

Floru, L., Ishay, J., and Gitter, S. The influence of psychotropic substances on hornet behavior in colonies of *Vespa orientalis F*. (Hymenoptera). *Psychopharmacologia*, 1969, **14**, 323–341.

Frankenhaeuser, M., Post, B., Hagdahl, R., and Wrangsjoe, B. Effects of a depressant drug as modified by experimentally-induced expectation. *Perceptual and Motor Skills*, 1964, **18**, 513–522.

Frankenhaeuser, M., Myrsten, A.-L., Post, B., and Johansson, G. Behavioral and physiological effects of cigarette smoking in a monotonous situation. *Psychopharmacologia*, 1971, **22**, 1–7.

Freund, J., Krupp, G., Goodenough, D., and Preston, L. W. The doctor-patient relationship and drug effect. *Clinical Pharmacology and Therapeutics*, 1972, **13**, 172–180.

Gaddum, J. H. and Hameed, K. A. Drugs which antagonize 5-hydroxytryptamine. *British Journal of Pharmacology and Chemotherapy*, 1954, **9**, 240–248.

Goodman, L. S. and Gilman, A. *The pharmacological basis of therapeutics*, 4th ed. London: Macmillan, 1970.

Gottschalk, L. A. The measurement of hostile aggression through the content analysis of speech. In S. Garattini and E. B. Sigg (Eds.), *Aggressive behavior*. New York: Wiley, 1969.

Gottschalk, L. A., Gleser, G. C., Stone, W. N., and Kunkel R. L. Studies of psychoactive drug effects on nonpsychiatric patients: Measurement of affective and cognitive changes by content analysis of speech. In W. O. Evans and N. S. Kline (Eds.), *The psychopharmacology of the normal human*. Springfield: Charles C. Thomas, 1969.

Haward, L. R. C. Differential modifications of verbal aggression by psychotropic drugs. In S. Garattini and E. B. Sigg (Eds.), *Aggressive behavior*. New York: Wiley, 1969.

Health, Education, and Welfare, Department of. *Smoking and Health, Report of the Advisory Committee to the Surgeon General of the Public Health Service.* (USPHS Rep. No. 1103) Washington, D. C.: U.S. Government Printing Office, 1964.

Herrington, R. N. The effect of amphetamine on a serial reaction task. *Psychopharmacologia,* 1967, **12,** 50–57.

Hill, H. E., Belleville, R. E., and Wikler, A. Motivational determinants in modification of behavior by morphine and pentobarbital. *Archives of Neurology and Psychiatry,* 1957, **77,** 28–35.

Hofmann, A. Psychotomimetic drugs: chemical and pharmacological aspects. *Acta Physiologica et Pharmacologica Neelandica,* 1959, **8,** 240–258.

Höhn, R. and Lasagna, L. Effects of aggregation and temperature on amphetamine toxicity in mice. *Psychopharmacologia,* 1960, **1,** 210–220.

Hornbein, T. F. *Everest–the west ridge.* New York: Ballantine, 1968.

Hornykiewicz, O. Dopamine (3-hydroxytryptamine) and brain function. *Pharmacological Reviews,* 1966, **18,** (2), 925–964.

Hunt, W. A. and Matarazzo, J. D. Three years later: recent developments in the experimental modification of smoking behavior. *Journal of Abnormal Psychology,* 1973, **81**(2), 107–114.

Huxley, A. *The doors of perception.* New York: Harper & Brothers, 1954.

Jaattela, A., Mannisto, P., Paatero, H., and Tuomisto, J. The effects of diazepam or diphenhydramine on healthy human subjects. *Psychopharmacologia,* 1971, **21,** 202–211.

Jarvik, M. E. Drugs used in the treatment of psychiatric disorders. In E. S. Goodman and A. Gilman (Eds.), *The pharmacological basis of therapeutics,* 4th ed. New York: Macmillan, 1970. *(a)*

Jarvik, M. E. The role of nicotine in the smoking habit. In W. A. Hunt (Ed.), *Learning mechanisms in smoking.* Chicago: Aldine, 1970. *(b)*

Johannsen, D. E. Perception. In P. R. Farnsworth (Ed.), *Annual review of psychology.* Palo Alto: Annual Reviews, 1967.

Johnson, F. N. Chlorpromazine and lithium. *Disease of the Nervous System,* 1972, **33,** 235–241.

Jones, R. Marijuana-induced "high": Influence of expectation, setting and previous drug experience. *Pharmacological Reviews,* 1971, **23,** 359–369.

Joyce, C. R. B. Experiments with control substances. *Annals of the Rheumatic Diseases,* 1961, **20,** 78–82.

Joyce, C. R. B. Placebo reactions. In P. Hopkins and H. H. Wolff (Eds.), *Principles of treatments of psychosomatic disorders.* London: Pergamon, 1965.

Joyce, C. R. B. Can drugs affect personality? In I. T. Ramsey and R. Porter (Eds.), *Personality and science.* London: Churchill Livingston, 1971.

Kane, F. J., Jr., Lipton, M. A., Krall, A. R., and Obrist, P. A. Psychoendocrine study of oral contraceptive agents. *American Journal of Psychiatry,* 1970, **127,** 85–92.

Knapp, P., Bliss, C. M., and Wells, H. Addictive aspects in heavy cigarette smoking. *American Journal of Psychiatry,* 1963, **119,** 966–972.

Korf, J. and Kuiper, H. E. Induction of bizarre behavior in rats by p-chloramphetamine, a serotonin depletor, after repeated drug administration. *Psychopharmacologia*, 1971, **21**, 328–337.

Krsiak, M., Borgesova, M., and Kadlecova, O. LSD accentuated individual type of social behavior in mice. *Activitas Nervosa Superior*, 1971, **13**, 211–212.

Kubzansky, P. E. The effects of reduced environmental stimulation on human behavior: a review. In A. D. Biderman and H. Zimmer (Eds.), *The manipulation of human behavior*. New York: Wiley, 1961.

Kuhn, R. The treatment of depressive states with G22355 (imipramine hydrochloride). *American Journal of Psychiatry*, 1958, **115**, 459–464.

Latz, A. Cognitive test performance of normal human adults under the influence of psychopharmacological agents: A brief review. In D. H. Efron (Ed.), *Psychopharmacology, a review of progress 1957–1967*. (USPHS pub. No. 1836) Washington, D. C.: U.S. Government Printing Office, 1968.

Leary, T. *High priest*. New York: World, 1968.

Lehmann, H. E. and Knight, M. A. Placebo-proneness and placebo resistance of different psychological functions. *Psychiatric Quarterly*, 1960, **34**, 505–516.

Lehrman, D. S. Control of behavior cycles in reproduction. In W. Etkin (Ed.), *Social behavior and organization among vertebrates*. Chicago: University of Chicago Press, 1964.

Lennard, H. L., Epstein, L. J., Bernstein, A. and Ransom, D. C. *Mystification and drug misuse*. San Francisco: Jossey-Bass, Inc. 1971.

Lucchesi, B. R., Schuster, C. R., and Emley, G. S. The role of nicotine as a determinant of cigarette smoking frequency in man with observations of certain cardiovascular effects associated with the tobacco alkaloid. *Clinical Pharmacology and Therapeutics*, 1967, **8**, 789–796.

Maas, J. W., Fawcett, J., and Dekirmenjian, H. 3-Methoxy-4-hydroxyphenylglycol (MHPG) excretion in depressive states. *Archives of General Psychiatry*, 1968, **19**, 129–134.

Masur, J., Martz, R. M. W., and Carlini, E. A. The behavior of worker and non-worker rats under the influence of (-)$\Delta^9$-transtetraphydrocannabinol, chlorpromazine and amylobarbitone. *Psychopharmacologia*, 1972, **25**, 57–68.

McClearn, G. E. The genetic aspects of alcoholism. In P. G. Bourne and R. Fox (Eds.), *Alcoholism–progress in research and treatment*. New York: Academic, 1973.

McGaugh, J. L. Drug facilitation of memory and learning. In D. Efron (Ed.), *Psychopharmacology: A review of progress*. (USPHS Pub. No. 1836) Washington, D. C.: U.S. Government Printing Office, 1968.

Miller, N. E. Effects of drugs on motivation: The value of using a variety of measures. *Annals of the New York Academy of Sciences*, 1956, **65**, 318–333.

Myrsten, A.-L., Andersson, K., Frankenhaeuser, M., and Mardh, A. Immediate effects of cigarette smoking as related to different smoking habits. *Report of the Psychological Laboratory*, University of Stockholm, No. 378, 1972.

Myrsten, A.-L., Post, B., Frankenhaeuser, M., and Johansson, G. Changes in behavioral and physiological activation induced by cigarette smoking in habitual smokers. *Psychopharmacologia*, 1972, **27**, 305–318.

Nowlis, V. and Nowlis, H. H. The description and analysis of mood. *Annals of the New York Academy of Sciences*, 1956, **65**, 345–356.

Porsolt, R. D., Joyce, D., and Summerfield, A. Changes in behavior with repeated testing under the influence of drugs: Drug-experience interactions. *Nature*, 1970, **227**, 286–287.

Porte, D., Jr. and Robertson, R. P. Control of insulin secretion by catecholamines, stress, and the sympathetic nervous system. *Federation Proceedings*, 1973, **32**, 1792–1796.

Randrup, A. and Munkvad, I. Relation of brain catecholamines to aggressiveness and other forms of behavioral excitation. In S. Garattini and E. B. Sigg (Eds.), *Aggressive behavior*. New York: Wiley, 1969.

Redmond, D. E., Jr., Hinrichs, R. L., Maas, J. W., and Kling, A. Behavior of free-ranging macaques after intraventricular 6-hydroxydopamine. *Science*, 1973, **181**, 1256–1258.

Redmond, D. E., Jr., Maas, J. W., Kling, A., and Dekirmenjian, H. Changes in primate social behavior after treatment with alpha-methyl-paratyrosine. *Psychosomatic Medicine*, 1971, **33**, 97–113.

Redmond, D. E., Jr., Maas, J. W., Kling, A., Graham, C. W., and Dekirmenjian, H. Social behavior of monkeys selectively depleted of monoamines. *Science*, 1971, **174**, 428–431.

Riklan M. An L-dopa paradox: Bipolar behavioral alterations. *Journal of the American Geriatrics Society*, 1972, **20**, 572–575.

Ross, S., Krugman, A. D., Lyerly, S. B., and Clyde, D. Drugs and placebos: a model design. *Psychological Reports*, 1962, **10**, 383–392.

Rothballer, A. Effects of catecholamines on the central nervous system. *Pharmacological Reviews*, 1959, **11**, 494–547.

Schachter, S. The interaction of cognitive and physiological determinants of emotional state. In P. H. Leiderman and D. Shapiro (Eds.), *Psychobiological approaches to social behavior*. Stanford: Stanford University Press, 1964.

Schildkraut, J. J. *Neuropsychopharmacology and the affective disorders*. Boston: Little, Brown, 1970.

Schlittler, E., MacPhillamy, H. B., Dorfman, L., Furlenmeier, A., Huebner, C. F., Lucas, R., Mueller, J. M., Schwyzer R., and Saint-Andre, A. F. Chemistry of rauwolfia alkaloids, including reserpine. *Annals of the New York Academy of Sciences*, 1954, **59**, 1–7.

Shou, M. Lithium in psychiatry, a review. In D. Efron (Ed.), *Psychopharmacology: A review of progress*. (USPHS Pub. No. 1836) Washington, D. C.: U.S. Government Printing Office, 1968.

Siegel, R. K. An ethologic search for self-administration of hallucinogens. *International Journal of the Addictions*, 1973, **8**, 373–393. *(a)*

Siegel, R. K. Visual imagery constants: Drug-induced changes in trained and untrained observers. *Proceedings, 81st Annual Convention, American Psychological Association*, 1973, 1033–1034. *(b)*

Slater, P. E. and Kastenbaum, R. Paradoxical reactions to drugs: some personality and ethnic correlates. *Journal of the American Geriatrics Society*, 1966, **14**, 1016–1034.

Starkweather, J. A. Individual and situational influences on drug effects. In R. M. Featherstone and A. Simon (Eds.), *A pharmacologic approach to the study of the mind*. Springfield: Charles C. Thomas, 1959.

Stoller, R. J. *Sex and gender*. New York: Science House, 1968.

Suedfeld, P. Changes in intellectual performance and in susceptibility to influence. In J. P. Zubek (Ed.), *Sensory deprivation: fifteen years of research*. New York: Appleton-Century-Crofts, 1969.

Talland, G. A. and Quarton, G. C. The effects of methamphetamine and pentobarbital on the running memory span. *Psychopharmacologia*, 1965, **7**, 379–382.

Talland, G. A. and Quarton, G. C. The effects of drugs and familiarity on performance in continuous visual search. *Journal of Nervous and Mental Disease*. 1966, **143**, 87–91.

Tikal, K. and Benesova, O. The effect of pyrithioxin (Encephabol Merck) on behavior, learning and biochemical variables of brain in rats malnourished in early life. II. Active avoidance and discriminative learning. *Activitas Nervosa Superior*, 1972, **14**, 174–175. (a)

Tikal, K. and Benesova, O. The effect of some psychotropic drugs on contact behavior in a group of rats. *Activitas Nervosa Superior*, 1972, **14**, 168–170. (b)

Thor, D. H. Amphetamine induced fighting during morphine withdrawal. *Journal of General Psychology*, 1971, **84**, 245–250.

Van der Poel, A. M. and Remmelts, M. The effect of anticholinergics on the behavior of the rat in a solitary and in a social situation. *Archives Internationales de Pharmacodynamie et de Therapie*, 1971, **189**, 394–396.

Vesell, E. S., Page, J. G., and Passananti, G. T. Genetic and environmental factors affecting ethanol metabolism in man. *Clinical Pharmacology and Therapeutics*, 1971, **12**, 192–201.

Vogel, J. R. and Leaf, R. C. Initiation of mouse killing in nonkiller rats by repeated pilocarpine treatment. *Physiology and Behavior*, 1972, **8**, 421–424.

Vojtechovsky, M., Safratova, V., and Havrankova, O. Effect of threshold doses of lysergic acid diethylamide (LSD) on social interaction in healthy students. *Activitas Nervosa Superior*, 1972, **14**, 115–116.

Weihe, W. H. The effect of temperature on the action of drugs. In H. W. Elliott (Ed.), *Annual Review of Pharmacology*, 1973, **13**, 409–425.

Weiss, B. and Laties, V. G. Enhancement of human performance by caffeine and the amphetamines. *Pharmacological Reviews*, 1962, **14**, 1–36.

Welch, B. L. Symposium summary. In S. Garattini and E. B. Sigg (Eds.), *Aggressive behavior*. New York: Wiley, 1969.

Whalen, R. E. Sexual motivation. *Psychological Review*, 1966, **73**, 151–163.

Wikler, A. Interaction of physical dependence, classical and operant conditioning in the genesis of relapse. In A. Wikler (Ed.), *The addictive states*. Baltimore: Williams and Wilkins, 1968.

Wolf, S., Doering, C. R., Clark, M. L., and Hagans, J. A. Chance distribution and the placebo "reactor." *Journal of Laboratory and Clinical Medicine,* 1957, **49,** 837–841.

Zuckerman, M. Hallucinations, reported sensations and images. In J. P. Zubek (Ed.), *Sensory deprivation: Fifteen years of research.* New York: Appleton-Century-Crofts, 1969.

CHAPTER 2

# Evaluating the Therapeutic Effects of Psychoactive Drugs by Sociopsychological Methods*

RICHARD L. COOK

The rapid proliferation of therapeutic uses of psychoactive drugs during the last two decades began with the serendipitous discovery of chlorpromazine, a drug with new major tranquilizing effects (Gershon, 1970). As a result of this discovery, approximately 85% of patients in mental hospitals in the United States are currently being given psychoactive medication, and hundreds of thousands of outpatients are being treated with them as well. But the interactions between patient, diagnosis, drug, and situational variables remain poorly understood. Moreover, many, if not all, psychiatrists and psychologists would agree with Hollister's contention that the abundance of psychotherapeutic drugs has contributed "... more to the confusion of physicians than to benefits for patients [1972a, p. 984]." Hollister (1972a, 1972b) also suggests that comparative studies have failed to clarify the situation, inasmuch as little difference in efficacy has been demonstrated between various antipsychotic drugs, and, indeed, there is minimal evidence for any advantage of antianxiety and antidepressant drugs over a placebo. (Further evidence on this issue is presented in Chapters 4, 5, 7, 8, 9, 10, 11, and 12 of this volume.)

The wide use of drugs having biochemical and behavioral consequences that are even now not completely clear, poses, or should pose, a medical and psychological problem if for no other reason than that such drugs have serious side effects (see, e.g., Crane, 1973).

*Preparation of this paper was aided by bibliographic searches provided by the National Institute of Mental Health, the MEDLARS service of the National Library of Medicine, and the Primate Information Center at the University of Washington.

It is the contention of this paper that the inability to discover many important behavioral consequences of psychoactive drugs is due to the use of inadequate psychological methods for assessing drug effects. Krech (1972) argues that although researchers in the field of biochemistry and behavior know much about biochemistry and physiology, they often remain unsophisticated in their approach to behavior, an asymmetry which has produced what he calls "half-assessed experiments." Manipulations of chemical structure yield promising new psychoactive compounds, but traditional psychological assessment methodology does not adequately indicate to what extent behavior is changed.

Traditional assessment methodology has proved inadequate for this task (see Newmark, 1971) because it is only indirectly related to important dimensions of behavior. Since social behavior is what therapeutic drugs are intended to improve, one ultimate criterion must be to improve social functioning in situations outside the institution. But social behavior is not the central focus of traditional assessment methods; it is assessed only indirectly and imprecisely.

This review proceeds in the following way: first, the failures of traditional methods to differentiate between psychoactive drugs are discussed; second, the rationale for considering improved social functioning as the primary criterion for patient improvement is given; third, some research techniques from the field of social psychology that show considerable promise for providing direct assessment of the effects of psychoactive drugs on social behavior are described.

## INADEQUACIES OF TRADITIONAL ASSESSMENT METHODOLOGY

Traditional psychometric methods of assessment involve the use of psychological tests, such as the Minnesota Multiphasic Personality Inventory (MMPI), and a variety of rating scales, such as the Inpatient Multidimensional Psychiatric Scale (IMPS), behavioral and prognostic rating scales, mood, personality, and attitudinal scales, and so on (see Grayson, 1970). Most of these rely on a clinician's interview with the patient although some involve behavioral ratings by nurses or other hospital personnel or, less frequently, self-ratings.

Although such psychometric measures have occasionally yielded positive results in studies of psychoactive drug effects, failures in cross-validation studies have been frequent. For example, Goldberg, Mattsson, Cole, and Klerman (1967) used multiple regression techniques to demonstrate that specific pretreatment symptom patterns were associated with improvement under each of four different phenothiazines. Results for two of the drugs, chlorpromazine and fluphenazine, were cross-validated. Goldberg and Mattsson (1968) factor analyzed the 21 independent variables and obtained six second-order factors and extended the analysis to include a demonstration of the prediction pattern for improvement on placebo.

However, when Goldberg, Frosch, Drossman, Schooler, and Johnson (1972) attempted to use these multiple regression equations to predict response to acetophenazine and chlorpromazine with a new sample of patients, they were unsuccessful. These authors discuss the failures and successes of other attempts to cross-validate similar findings; they suggest that, while the positive results cannot be lightly dismissed, the hypothesis of differential responding to these two phenothiazines remains unproven.

Forsythe, May, and Engelman discuss the statistical difficulties of attempting to obtain a multiple regression equation that would be useful in cross-validation studies and suggest alternative procedures (May & Forsythe, 1970; Forsythe, May, & Engelman, 1970, 1971). Klett, one of the developers of the Inpatient Multidimensional Psychiatric Scale, a 75-item rating scale based on interview behavior (Lorr, Klett, McNair, & Lasky, 1963), has suggested that although the prevailing methodology may prove to be satisfactory for screening active agents from a placebo, it does not discriminate between active agents (Klett, 1968). Klett considered a number of widely used rating scales in reaching this conclusion (the IMPS, the Wittenborn Psychiatric Rating Scale, the Brief Psychiatric Rating Scale, and the Psychotic Reaction Profile).

A recently introduced psychometric approach uses symptom clusters to differentiate between patient responses to treatment, rather than relying on diagnostic subgroups (Goldstein, Brauzer, & Caldwell, 1970). For example, Klein, Feldman, and Honigfeld (1970) maintain that univariate, global improvement, total morbidity, composite, and factor scores all fail to depict distinct patterns of drug-induced change. They propose that behavioral changes in patients can be more effectively described if patterns of change are specified, and Klein and his colleagues have shown that their method demonstrates both drug effects and diagnosis-drug interactions.

Other new psychometric procedures emphasize social behavior more than do traditional pathological indicators such as the MMPI (Trott & Morf, 1972) and the Differential Personality Inventory (DPI). The latter also appears to be psychometrically superior to the MMPI (Jackson & Carlson, 1969).

Recent psychometric approaches to the assessment of mental illness represent a trend towards rejection of the disease model implicit in the concept of "mental illness." An influential, if controversial, critique of the disease model was given by Szasz (1961) in *The Myth of Mental Illness*. He and other writers have continued the attack on the mental illness "metaphor" (Sarbin, 1969) in both popular and scientific sources. Indeed, Albee (1968, 1973) has argued that the illness model has been used as an excuse for social repression, and has also resulted in the misallocation of mental health resources and manpower. Ranabauer (1968) even claims that clinicians have an emotional over-investment in diagnostic labels resulting from the role played by these variables in reducing cognitive strain and camouflaging a lack of information. The reports by "normal volunteers" who were admitted to mental hospitals (Rosenhan, 1973) vividly document the misuse and permanence of the label "schizophrenia" (see also Baruk, 1973, for a commentary on misuse of this popular label). Thus, many researchers have questioned the usefulness of traditional diagnostic classifications (see Phillips & Draguns, 1971, for a review of this trend).

The rejection of traditional diagnostic categories has been accompanied by an increased emphasis on the *social* aspects of mental illness (see Glidewell, 1972). Krasner goes so far as to argue that "Behavior changes only in a social context [Krasner, 1968, p. 171]," that what is referred to as mental illness might better be called "social disability" (see, for example, Vance, 1973). Ruesch and Brodsky (1968) believe that physical, psychological, and social impairment can all be subsumed by the concept of social disability. "Mental dysfunctioning" represents a less radical terminology but does avoid some of the unwarranted connotations of "mental illness."

The growing awareness that traditional methods of assessment are inadequate for demonstrating effects of psychoactive drugs has thus been accompanied by an acknowledgment of the need to consider more explicitly the social dimensions of mental dysfunctioning, as well as direct measures of social interaction and competence. Whether the results of future investigations will cause what is now called "mental illness" to be called "social disability" (Vance, 1973) remains to be seen. It cannot be doubted, however, that just as surely as efforts to understand the biochemical basis of psychological processes increase, so will efforts to understand the social basis of such processes.

## THE SOCIAL BASIS OF MENTAL DYSFUNCTIONING

In a recent comprehensive text on psychiatric treatment, Detre and Jarecki (1971) propose that social dysfunctioning is the common element in definitions of mental illness. They note that mental illness and social dysfunctioning tend to covary and they state that ". . . we consider an individual to have a psychiatric illness only when we see evidence of *social dysfunctioning* coupled with symp-

toms of *psychological and biological discomfort,* and believe that the dysfunctioning and discomfort are caused by disturbances in the mechanisms *that regulate
mood and cognition* [pp. 22–23, their italics].''

Detre and Jarecki reject the traditional, more inclusive, definitions of mental
illness as so broad as to be meaningless. They argue that the criterion of social
dysfunctioning offers the advantages of being readily observable, implying more
obvious norms, and avoiding the nebulous concept of an idealized state of mental
health. In particular, they suggest that three areas of social competency might be
taken as important determinants of the clinician's assessment of an individual's
mental health: interactions with one's family, interactions with one's peers, and
the successful pursuit of an occupation. Interpersonal learning on both emotional
and cognitive levels is basic to Detre and Jarecki's argument. Research in the
setting of a mental hospital should be designed to investigate *directly* how emotional and cognitive functioning relates to *interpersonal* behavior; the more direct
such measures are, the more successful they are likely to be.

The importance of social interaction in mental health is attested to by a growing
number of researchers. For example, in a recent study of hospitalized schizophrenic patients, Klein, Person, and Itil (1972) found that recent social events and
such social factors as family behavior were significantly related to clinical outcome whereas the number of times hospitalized and length of hospital stay were
not. Goldberg and his colleagues (1972) also consider that hospitalization is now
less associated with dramatic symptomatology than with social failure; patients are
now being rated as less severely ill than formerly. They indicate that whether or
not this change explains their failure to cross-validate earlier results, alternative
methods for assessing mental dysfunctioning are clearly needed.

## CONTRIBUTIONS OF SOCIAL PSYCHOLOGY

The increasing interest in social aspects of mental dysfunctioning, together with
the generally recognized need for better methods for the description and measurement of the effects of psychoactive drugs, suggests that research methods drawn
from social psychology for the direct assessment of drug effects on social interaction may be useful.

The goal of the following sections is a representative overview, not a comprehensive review of the methods of social psychology. Having shown that social
interaction is now considered to be important in assessing patient functioning, the
remainder of the chapter describes research methods that seem most relevant. Bias
in the selection of the methods reflects the author's background, but does not affect

the overall conclusion: certain research methods of social psychology have considerable potential for adding to our understanding of the effects of drugs but are underutilized at the present time.

The general reviews of each topic noted, and specific references to studies demonstrating the use of the methods in investigations of drug effects may be supplemented by the more comprehensive treatments in *The Handbook of Social Psychology* edited by Lindzey and Aronson (5 vols., 1968–1969) and the textbook by McClintock (1972). The handbook of empirical studies of behavior change and psychotherapy edited by Bergin and Garfield (1971), which includes the review by Goldstein and Simonson (1971), also contains a number of informative chapters. Other major sources include collected papers on psychoactive drugs edited by May and Wittenborn (1969) and Wittenborn, Goldberg, and May (1970), and others on assessment edited by McReynolds (1968, 1971).

The next section discusses (1) some systematic techniques for observing and categorizing the elements of social interaction, (2) experimental designs intended to standardize and simplify the setting in which the interaction occurs, and (3) experimental research paradigms derived from theoretical descriptions of the nature of social interaction.

## SYSTEMATIC OBSERVATION OF SOCIAL INTERACTION

Good observational methods are those that systematically record behavior. This definition is purposely broad and clearly includes such frequently used devices as the behavioral rating scales discussed earlier. But the methodology of systematic observation (Weick, 1968) has been extensively developed by social psychologists, and many of the observational techniques could be quite useful to researchers studying the effects of drugs on patient interaction.

It is important to note that a systematic observation need not be passive observation, although unobtrusive measures can often be devised and should prove useful in many situations (Webb, Campbell, Schwartz, & Sechrest, 1966). Weick (1968), who has reviewed the use of observational techniques by social psychologists, believes that systematic observation would often benefit from some degree of direct experimental manipulation. For example, subjects receiving different drugs might participate in structured discussions or tasks, their behavior being observed and recorded.

Specific techniques for recording behavior are described below.

and notes that aspects picked up by the "cloze" procedure, as well as vocal characteristics of speech and pausing behavior, appear to be least affected by situational variables. He suggests that speech behavior should therefore be a more sensitive indicator of internal influences, such as drugs. But in her review of experimental studies of drug effects on speech, Waskow (1967a) cautions that "At the present time it is impossible to attempt a theoretical integration of the results of these studies. They are too few, and the differences among them and their methodological weaknesses are too great for any valid conclusions to be drawn [p. 356]." This would still be true in 1974. The methods for studying verbal and related phenomena show considerable promise for the study of drug influence on social interaction. The fulfillment of this promise depends upon the systematic application of these methods within the context of better theories about social behavior.

## Physiological Correlates of Interaction

Physiological variables are unquestionably affected by social interaction, but this field of research is quite new, and findings are limited as yet (see Shapiro and Crider, 1969). The cumbersome equipment previously needed for recording physiological responses prevented systematic observation in circumstances resembling normal social interaction, but has been improved by electronic miniaturization. "With the advent of telemetry, it has become possible to monitor the patient's state as he goes about his daily activities [Frank, 1968, p. 50]." The refinement of such methodological innovations can be expected to lead to theoretical advances in specifying relationships between physiological and social variables. New instruments may become even more valuable as the theoretical relations between physiological and psychological variables are clarified so that the physiological measures decided upon can be made appropriate to the social context.

## Social Behavior of Infrahuman Subjects

Although not a technique in the sense used above, the systematic observation of the social behavior of infrahuman subjects (Zajonc, 1969; Scott, 1969; Chance, 1968) is a field of social psychological research that could yield useful information about the effects of psychoactive drugs. Studies of such effects are instructive, and some are therefore described below (see also Chapter 1 of this book).

Lister, Beattie, and Berry (1971) studied established colonies of baboons and produced anxiety and aggression in the colony leader by such techniques as having a human enter the cage. Social and other behaviors of the baboons were rated and the leader was then given various drugs. These authors concluded that "Pentobarbital and chlorpromazine appeared to reduce anxiety and aggression by producing a form of sedation. Medazepam in contrast not only reduced anxiety and aggression, but 'released' the animal to permit it to behave normally, particularly as far as eating, drinking and social interactions were concerned [pp. 302–303]."

Schiørring and Randrup (1971) and Kjellberg and Randrup (1971) have demonstrated experimentally the critical importance of assessing changes in social behavior when drug effects are considered, and indicate the implications of their findings for research with humans.

Since infrahuman subjects are used to evaluate drug effects, their social behavior should be studied. Of course, cross-species generalizations should not be carried too far, but experiments with infrahuman subjects in social situations could provide useful ways to gather preliminary evidence about the effects of drugs (see Miller, Levine, & Mirsky, 1973), as well as to generate hypotheses to be studied subsequently in human subject populations.

## Comment on Observational Methodology

The subtle interrelations of verbal and related behavioral events can be seen in the discussion by Murray and Jacobson (1971) of the analysis of interaction as communication at several levels by Haley (1963): words, vocal and linguistic patterns, bodily movements, and the context in which these take place. Haley sees these behaviors as attempts to communicate which may be either congruent or dissonant with each other. Murray and Jacobson (1971) consider the application of such concepts to psychoanalysis and desensitization, and conclude that Haley's novel conceptions demonstrate that "An adequate model of social learning in psychotherapy will have to deal directly with the interpersonal meaning of behavior [p. 741]."

Combinations of observational methods will probably be most fruitful in the investigation of the complexities of such behavior. Lanyon (1971), for example, has advocated the systematic application of a "technology" of mental health which would include automation of many of the routine aspects of assessment, using computers to administer, score, and interpret traditional assessment devices and possibly to collect data using a number of the observational techniques that have been reviewed. This procedure would free the clinician from some routine activities and provide him with a broader base for his judgments, but of course it would by no means be accepted by psychiatrists throughout the world.

## CONTROLLED OBSERVATIONAL SETTINGS

The discussion of observational methods has emphasized techniques ordinarily used to study relatively spontaneous behavior in naturalistic settings. Social psychologists have also used a variety of controlled experimental or observational settings to study rather straightforward variables, such as a player's bid in a bargaining game.

### Experimental Games

A vast number of structured activities may qualify as "games" but game theory is based on a rather special sort of interaction between (usually) two "players." English and English (1958) define this as "... a mathematical theory that deals with action in a conflict situation as if it were a game in which each player seeks to maximize his opponents' losses. The player is assumed to be a wholly rational being, utilizing calculations of risk [p. 220]." In fact, however, these assumptions do not lead to realistic predictions of behavior, even by normal persons, and such narrow definitions have limited the exploitation of a potentially valuable research technique. Researchers involved in the study of human behavior have tended to assume that experimental games were inextricably bound up with unrealistic expectations of player rationality.

In the type of game referred to, two players make one or more choices, or moves, and receive rewards or punishments (money or points, for example) that are determined by the moves of both players. The result of any combination of moves by the players can be described by a "payoff" matrix. Depending on the payoff matrix, such games may be either purely competitive (zero-sum) or cooperative (mixed-motive). Some different kinds of game studies, as well as the logic of game theory, are described in Luce and Raiffa (1957) and Rapoport (1966).

However, experimental games need not be viewed simply as techniques for demonstrating the failure of human rationality, nor do the research needs of the psychologist have to be overshadowed by the proofs of the mathematician. Games can also be seen as evoking significant examples of human interaction, in which important aspects of patient functioning such as cooperation, conflict, hostility, reciprocation, and so forth, occur within a well-defined and controlled setting. Rapoport (1969) believes that "The principal advantage of the game method in psychological research lies in the circumstance that, while the thought processes so tapped are quite rich in psychological content . . ., the experimental tool itself is an extremely simple one [p. 139]."

Game theory is only beginning to be fruitfully applied to realistic situations involving meaningful dimensions of behavior, a focus requiring the development of more sophisticated statistical measures of behavioral change during the game. For example, Harris (1971) discusses the uses of games in personality research, and suggests that measures of intra-individual changes during the course of a game or games must be found.

Some effects of psychoactive drugs on game behavior were demonstrated by Hurst, Radlow, Chubb, and Bagley (1969). Subjects given a placebo, $d$-amphetamine, amobarbital, or a combination of the two drugs participated in a series of mixed-motive games to win substantial amounts of money (as much as $45.00!) Amphetamine affected measures indicative of style of play, although not of overall game performance, that could not be predicted from self-ratings of mood.

Other games studied by psychologists differ in format from the games described above, but the concepts are similar. For example, Deutsch has examined cooperation and conflict in a game requiring two players to coordinate their game strategies for either player to benefit (Deutsch, 1969; Deutsch & Krauss, 1962). The game requires players to control the route followed by a truck, with routes and movements displayed on a board. An important advantage of the game is that the experimental procedure is interesting to the participants. At a slightly more complex level there are experimental games with three or more participants. A number of authors have noted that these are distinct from the games discussed above because two or more players can form a coalition (Gamson, 1964; Caplow, 1956) and thus bring another important social process under scrutiny.

## Simulations

Although the games above described may be played under relatively realistic conditions, most experiments using them have tended to be highly artificial (Avedon & Sutton-Smith, 1971). Laboratory games could be made much more realistic and interesting and still retain the advantages of studying social interaction in relatively well controlled settings, such as those provided by simulations. These may be seen as complex games involving structured interaction in realistic situations. Although currently available simulations might be used as settings for patient interaction, simulations of business operations or of tasks related to those patients might face could be devised. Observational techniques would be used to assess the ability of the patient to function effectively in occupational and other settings. Simulations might also be therapeutic for participants.

Theories of social interaction can be considerably improved through the appropriate use of the techniques of gaming and simulation (see Raser, Campbell, & Chadwick, 1970). Experimental games and simulations represent realistic, but structured, situations involving interpersonal learning and conflict that also allow for experimental manipulations (Boocock & Schild, 1968).

## RESEARCH PARADIGMS

Previous sections have focused on methods used in social psychology that might be used to study psychoactive drug effects. The next sections describe research based on theoretical developments in social psychology supported by a consistent body of empirical findings. The paradigms considered here are related to interpersonal learning, the ability of one person to learn *from* and *about* another person. Interpersonal learning is, of course, a critical aspect of effective functioning in a social setting, and should therefore also help to understand the effect of psychoactive drugs.

Murray and Jacobson (1971) comment that psychotherapy has come to be seen as a learning process by an increasing number of therapists in recent years, a point of view supported by Howard and Orlinsky (1972) in reviewing the function of the therapeutic system. They conclude that the major *de facto* function of psychotherapy apparently is to educate the patient in developing interpersonal skills as well as emotional stability. The personal distress that leads a patient to psychotherapy is "... occasioned by experienced frustration or failure in social-emotional functioning [p. 658]." The effect of psychotherapy is to educate the person so that he can correct the dysfunctional interpersonal and emotional patterns that have been learned. Possible interactions of drugs with such learning are clearly worth studying.

### Operant Conditioning and Social Reinforcers

Operant conditioning in social situations represents interpersonal learning at a simplistic level, but permits effective control of experimental conditions. Weiss

(1968) has reviewed the relevance of operant conditioning techniques to general questions of psychological assessment. He maintains that responsiveness to social reinforcers may be seen as an analogue (or sample) of behavior relevant to other interpersonal contexts and may be considered as a predictor (or sign) of other interpersonal behaviors. He suggests that "... we might profitably view behavior in the context of task demands and thus sample a wide range of adjustive behaviors [p. 174]." Weiss believes operant methodology is an appropriate assessment tool because it reflects important situational variables more clearly than do traditional assessment devices.

Krasner (1968, 1971) agrees with these conclusions in discussing the generalization of conditioning from one task to another. Thus, in one unpublished study mentioned by Krasner (1968), verbal conditioning in a laboratory task generalized to responsiveness to "token economy" reinforcements in the ward. However, although Lemaine and Guimelchain (1971) found only limited evidence for generalization of verbal conditioning, they emphasize the interest of verbal conditioning because of its obvious implications for understanding patient-therapist interactions.

Differential responsiveness to conditioning procedures, using social reinforcers, might well be used to study drug effects. An advantage of the technique is that both intra-individual and inter-individual changes could be assessed. Social reinforcers can also be expected to yield important information about drug effects on elementary dimensions of social behavior. Gupta (1973), for example, was able to demonstrate differential effects of dexedrine, phenobarbitone, ephedrine, and chlorpromazine on verbal conditioning for introverted and extroverted subjects.

### Modeling of Behavior

Modeling, the acquisition of a response by one person as a result of observing the responses of another, is concerned with more complex behavioral modification. The behavior acquired from models varies from simple responses to complex social dispositions, and in the context of therapy the process may be seen as one of social-emotional education. Modeling need not involve two-way interaction; it includes the observation of role models on television and in movies. Modeling plays an obvious role in the acculturation of children, but is undoubtedly an important determinant of adult behavior as well.

In a recent review of modeling and psychotherapy, Bandura (1971) summarizes

". . . three broad areas of psychological functioning in which modeling principles and treatment procedures . . . apply. These include the utilization of models to transmit new patterns of behavior, to eliminate unwarranted fears and inhibitions, and to facilitate expression of pre-existing modes of response [p. 703]." An examination of the influences of drugs on complex modeled behaviors would require sophisticated observational techniques. For example, patient role playing, a form of social imitation that could well be used more often in therapy (Davies, 1972), might be observed in the context of a structured simulation.

## Cognitive Aspects of Interpersonal Learning

The earlier discussion established the relevance of social interaction to an understanding of the effects of psychoactive drugs. The cognitive aspects of such interaction were emphasized by the review of Murray and Jacobson (1971): "The process of transmitting information . . . occurs in all forms of psychotherapy. . . . It appears that the role of informational learning has not been adequately emphasized, particularly with regard to the study of interpersonal behavior [p. 737]." An examination of cognitive dimensions of interaction complements the emphasis of Bandura (1969) and others on social learning.

Human judgment is the explicit focus of the research paradigm developed by Hammond and his associates. Hammond argues that the purely cognitive aspects of social interaction have been grossly underestimated in comparison with putative subconscious motivational and emotional factors. He describes in Chapter 3 the circumstances in which the processes of human judgment and their effect on interpersonal conflict and interpersonal learning may be studied.

Judgment is assumed to involve the process of combining uncertain information from a variety of sources in order to reach a decision about a state of affairs not wholly or immediately susceptible to scientific analysis. The weather forecaster, the stockbroker, for example, are professional "judges" or decision makers. But all of us make judgments frequently and in a variety of ways, and it is when such judgments are not modified by learning from and about others that troubles arise.

Hammond has developed experimental procedures for studying judgment as well as mathematical analyses of the judgment process (Hursch, Hammond, & Hursch, 1964; Hammond & Summers, 1972; see also Chapter 3 in this book). Judgmental learning tasks should help to understand the effect of drugs on social interaction. The method is probably unique in its explicit emphasis on the cognitive aspects of interpersonal processes.

## CONCLUSION

Mental dysfunction is expressed in part by problems in social interaction and interpersonal learning, yet traditional assessment devices deal only indirectly with social competence. This contradictory situation may well explain the inadequacies of these assessment techniques for determining the effects of psychoactive drugs. However, more and more investigators are becoming dissatisfied with this state of affairs. Peterson (1968), for example, rejected traditional research procedures and concluded that the individual should be viewed, and assessed, as a set of competencies.

As Elkes has put it in a discussion paraphrased in Smythies (1971): "As long as investigators fall back on the traditional procedure of trying to fit old nosologies to experimentally induced syndromes, there cannot be much progress. We should not be beguiled . . . by old names and must get away from a clinical 'model' for toxic psychoses. Let us look at the phenomena, at what these drugs can do, and try to codify the phenomena. A new nosology should be based on quantitative measurement of the degree of disorganization of disparate functions [p. 9–10]."

## REFERENCES

Albee, G. W. Conceptual models and manpower requirements in psychology. *American Psychologist*, 1968, **23**, 317–320.

Albee, G. W. Open letter to all concerned psychologists. *Society for the Psychological Study of Social Issues Newsletter*, 1973, **133**, 5.

Avedon, E. M. and Sutton-Smith, B. *The study of games.* New York: Wiley, 1971.

Bales, R. F. *Interacton process analysis.* Reading, Mass.: Addison-Wesley, 1950.

Bales, R. F. *Personal and interpersonal behavior.* New York: Holt, Rinehart & Winston, 1970.

Bandura, A. *Principles of behavior modification.* New York: Holt, Rinehart & Winston, 1969.

Bandura, A. Psychotherapy based upon modeling principles. In A. E. Bergin and S. L. Garfield (Eds.), *Handbook of psychotherapy and behavior change: An empirical analysis.* New York: Wiley, 1971.

Baruk, H. La revision de la schizophrenie. *Encèphale*, 1973, **62**, 56–77.

Bergin, A. E. and Garfield, S. L. (Eds.), *Handbook of psychotherapy and behavior change: An empirical analysis.* New York: Wiley, 1971.

Boocock, S. S. and Schild, E. O. *Simulation games in learning.* Beverly Hills: Sage, 1968.

Caplow, T. A theory of coalitions in the triad. *American Sociological Review*, 1956, **21**, 489–493.

Chance, M. R. A. Ethology and psychopharmacology. In C. R. B. Joyce (Ed.), *Psychopharmacology*. London: Tavistock, 1968.

Crane, G. E. Clinical psychopharmacology in its 20th year. *Science*, 1973, **181**, 124–128.

Davies, M. H. Social imitation: A neglected factor in psychotherapy. *British Journal of Psychiatry*, 1972, **121**, 281–285.

Detre, T. P. and Jarecki, H. G. *Modern psychiatric treatment*. Philadelphia: Lippincott, 1971.

Deutsch, M. Conflicts: Productive and destructive. *Journal of Social Issues*, 1969, **25**, 7–41.

Deutsch, M. and Krauss, R. M. Studies of interpersonal bargaining. *Journal of Conflict Resolution*, 1962, **6**, 52–76.

English, H. B. and English, A. C. *A comprehensive dictionary of psychological and psychoanalytical terms*. New York: David McKay, 1958.

Forsythe, A. B., May, P. R. A., and Engelman, L. Computing advantage scores by multiple regression. In J. R. Wittenborn and S. C. Goldberg (Eds.), *Psychopharmacology and the individual patient*. New York: Raven, 1970.

Forsythe, A. B., May, P. R. A., and Engelman, L. Prediction by multiple regression: How many variables to enter? *Journal of Psychiatric Research*, 1971, **8**, 119–126.

Frank, J. D. Methods of assessing the results of psychotherapy. In R. Porter (Ed.), *The role of learning in psychotherapy*. Boston: Little, Brown, 1968.

Gamson, W. Experimental studies of coalition formation. *Advances in Experimental Social Psychology*, 1964, **1**, 81–110.

Gershon, S. Predictiveness in psychopharmacology—preclinical-clinical correlations. In J. R. Wittenborn, S. C. Goldberg, and P. R. A. May (Eds.), *Psychopharmacology and the individual patient*. New York: Raven, 1970.

Glidewell, J. C. A social psychology of mental health. In S. E. Golann and C. Eisdorfer (Eds.), *Handbook of community mental health*. New York: Appleton-Century-Crofts, 1972.

Goldberg, S. C., Frosch, W. A., Drossman, A. K., Schooler, N. R., and Johnson, G. F. S. Prediction of response to phenothiazines in schizophrenia. *Archives of General Psychiatry*, 1972, **26**, 367–373.

Goldberg, S. C. and Mattsson, N. B. Schizophrenic sub-types defined by response to drugs and placebo. *Diseases of the Nervous System*, 1968, **29**, 153–158.

Goldberg, S. C., Mattsson, N. B., Cole, J. O., and Klerman, G. L. Prediction of improvement in schizophrenia under four phenothiazines. *Archives of General Psychiatry*, 1967, **16**, 107–117.

Goldman-Eisler, F. The relationship between temporal aspects of speech, the structure of language, and the state of the speaker. In K. Salzinger and S. Salzinger (Eds.), *Research in verbal behavior and some neurophysiological implications*. New York: Academic, 1967.

Goldstein, B. J., Brauzer, B., and Caldwell, J. M. The differential patterns of response to haloperidol and perphenazine. In J. R. Wittenborn, S. C. Goldberg, and P. R. A. May (Eds.), *Psychopharmacology and the individual patient*. New York: Raven, 1970.

Goldstein, A. P. and Simonson, N. R. Social psychological approaches to psychotherapy research. In A. E. Bergin and S. L. Garfield (Eds.), *Handbook of psychotherapy and behavior change: An empirical analysis*. New York: Wiley, 1971.

Gottschalk, L. A., Bates, D. E., Waskow, I. E., Katz, M. M., and Olsson, J. Effects of amphetamine or chlorpromazine on achievement striving scores derived from content analysis of speech. *Comprehensive Psychiatry*, 1971, **12**, 430–436.

Gottschalk, L. A. and Gleser, G. C. *The measurement of psychological states through the content analysis of verbal behavior*. Berkeley: University of California Press, 1969.

Gottschalk, L. A., Kapp, F. T., Ross, W. D., Kaplan, S. M., Silver, H., MacLeod, J. A., Kahn, J. B., Van Maanen, E. F., and Acheson, G. H. Explorations in testing drugs affecting physical and mental activity: Studies with a new drug of potential value in psychiatric illness. *Journal of the American Medical Association*, 1956, **161**, 1054–1058.

Grayson, H. M. Experimental design and assessment techniques in the clinical evaluation of psychotropic drugs. In W. G. Clark and J. del Giudice (Eds.), *Principles of psychopharmacology*. New York: Academic, 1970.

Gupta, B. S. The effects of stimulant and depressant drugs on verbal conditioning. *British Journal of Psychology*, 1973, **64**, 553–557.

Haley, J. *Strategies of psychotherapy*. New York: Grune and Stratton, 1963.

Hammond, K. R. and Summers, D. A. Cognitive control. *Psychological Review*, 1972, **79**, 58–67.

Harris, R. J. Experimental games as tools for personality research. In P. McReynolds (Ed.), *Advances in psychological assessment*. Vol. 2. Palo Alto: Science and Behavior Books, 1971.

Hollister, L. E. Mental disorders: Antipsychotic and antimanic drugs. *New England Journal of Medicine*, 1972, **286**, 984–987. *(a)*

Hollister, L. E. Mental disorders: Antianxiety and antidepressant drugs. *New England Journal of Medicine*, 1972, **286**, 1195–1198. *(b)*

Holsti, O. R. Content analysis. In G. Lindzey and E. Aronson (Eds.), *The handbook of social psychology*. Vol. 2, 2nd ed., Reading, Mass.: Addison-Wesley, 1968.

Honigfeld, G. Cloze analysis in the evaluation of central determinants of comprehensibility. In K. Salzinger and S. Salzinger (Eds.), *Research in verbal behavior and some neurophysiological implications*. New York: Academic, 1967.

Howard, K. I. and Orlinsky, D. E. Psychotherapeutic processes. *Annual Review of Psychology*, 1972, **23**, 615–668.

Hursch, C., Hammond, K. R., and Hursch, J. L. Some methodological considerations in multiple-cue probability studies. *Psychological Review*, 1964, **71**, 42–60.

Hurst, P. M., Radlow, R., Chubb, N., and Bagley, S. K. Drug effects upon behavior in mixed motive games. *Behavioral Science*, 1969, **14**, 443–452.

Jackson, D. N. and Carlson, K. A. Convergent and discriminant validation of the Differential Personality Inventory. *University of Western Ontario Research Bulletin*, No. 129, 1969.

Kjellberg, B. and Randrup, A. The effects of amphetamine and pimozide, a neuroleptic, on the social behavior of vervet monkeys (Cercopithecus Sp.). In O. Vinar, Z. Votava, and P. B. Bradley (Eds.), *Advances in neuropsychopharmacology*. Amsterdam: North-Holland, 1971.

Klein, D. F., Feldman, S., and Honigfeld, G. Can univariate measures of drug effect reflect clinical descriptions of change? In J. R. Wittenborn, S. C. Goldberg, and P. R. A. May (Eds.), *Psychopharmacology and the individual patient*. New York: Raven, 1970.

Klein, H., Person, T., and Itil, T. Family and environment variables as predictors of social outcome in chronic schizophrenia. *Comprehensive Psychiatry*, 1972, **13**, 317–334.

Klett, C. J. Assessing change in hospitalized psychiatric patients. In P. McReynolds (Ed.), *Advances in psychological assessment*. Vol. 1. Palo Alto: Science and Behavior Books, 1968.

Krasner, L. Assessment of token economy programmes in psychiatric hospitals. In R. Porter (Ed.), *Methods of assessing the results of psychotherapy*. Boston: Little, Brown, 1968.

Krasner, L. The operant approach in behavior therapy. In A. E. Bergin and S. L. Garfield (Eds.), *Handbook of psychotherapy and behavior change: An empirical analysis*. New York: Wiley, 1971.

Krech, D. Discussion. In J. L. McGaugh (Ed.), *The chemistry of mood, motivation, and memory*. New York: Plenum, 1972.

Lanyon, R. I. Mental health technology. *American Psychologist*, 1971, **26**, 1071–1076.

Lemaine, J. M. and Guimelchain, M. Conditionnement verbal et problémes cognitifs (1954–1969). *L'Année Psychologique*, 1971, **71**, 209–234.

Lindzey, G. and Aronson, E. (Eds.), *The handbook of social psychology*. 2nd ed., Reading, Mass.: Addison-Wesley, 1968–1969, 5 vols.

Lister, R. E., Beattie, I. A., and Berry, P. A. Effects of drugs on the social behavior of baboons. In O. Vinar, Z. Votava, and P. B. Bradley (Eds.), *Advances in neuro-psychopharmacology*. Amsterdam: North-Holland, 1971.

Lorr, M., Klett, C. J., McNair, D. M., and Lasky, J. J. *Inpatient multidimensional psychiatric scale manual*. Palo Alto: Consulting Psychologists Press, 1963.

Luce, R. D. and Raiffa, H. *Games and decisions*. New York: Wiley, 1957.

Marsden, G. Content-analysis studies of therapeutic interviews: 1954 to 1964. *Psychological Bulletin*, 1965, **63**, 298–321.

Marsden, G. Content analysis studies of psychotherapy: 1954 through 1968. In A. E. Bergin and S. L. Garfield (Eds.), *Handbook of psychotherapy and behavior change: An empirical analysis*. New York: Wiley, 1971.

May, P. R. A. and Forsythe, A. B. A contribution to the methodology of prediction: Advantage score technique. In J. R. Wittenborn and S. C. Goldberg (Eds.), *Psychopharmacology and the individual patient*. New York: Raven, 1970.

May, P. R. A. and Wittenborn, J. R. *Psychotropic drug response: Advances in prediction*. Springfield, Ill.: Charles C. Thomas, 1969.

McClintock, C. G. (Ed.), *Experimental social psychology*. New York: Holt, Rinehart & Winston, 1972.

McReynolds, P. (Ed.), *Advances in psychological assessment*. Vol. 1. Palo Alto: Science and Behavior Books, 1968.

McReynolds, P. (Ed.), *Advances in psychological assessment*. Vol. 2. Palo Alto: Science and Behavior Books, 1971.

Meurice, E. and Lemineur, R. Les essais d'approche objective et expérimentale des comportements de relation entre deux sujets (revue d'ensemble). *Encéphale*, 1971, **60**, 463–493.

Miller, R. E., Levine, J. M., and Mirsky, I. A. Effects of psychoactive drugs on nonverbal communication and group social behavior of monkeys. *Journal of Personality and Social Psychology*, 1973, **28**, 396–405.

Murray, E. J. and Jacobson, L. I. The nature of learning in traditional and behavioral psychotherapy. In A. E. Bergin and S. L. Garfield (Eds.), *Handbook of psychotherapy and behavior change: An empirical analysis*. New York: Wiley, 1971.

Newmark, C. S. Techniques used to assess the efficacy of psychotropic drugs: A critical review. *Psychological Reports*, 1971, **28**, 715–723.

Peterson, D. R. *The clinical study of social behavior*. New York: Appleton-Century-Crofts, 1968.

Phillips, L. and Draguns, J. G. Classification of the behavior disorders. *Annual Review of Psychology*, 1971, **22**, 447–482.

Ranabauer, W. Psychiatrishe Diagnosen unter psychologischen Gesichtspunkten. Nervenarzt, 1968, **39**, 205–213. Cited in L. Phillips and J. G. Draguns, Classification of the behavior disorders. *Annual Review of Psychology*, 1971, **22**, 447–482.

Rapoport, A. *Two-person game theory: The essential ideas*. Ann Arbor: University of Michigan Press, 1966.

Rapoport, A. Games as tools of psychological research. In I. R. Buchler and H. G. Nutini (Eds.), *Game theory in the behavioral sciences*. Pittsburgh: University of Pittsburgh Press, 1969.

Raser, J. R., Campbell, D. T., and Chadwick, R. W. Gaming and simulation for developing theory relevant to international relations. *General Systems*, 1970, **15**, 183–204.

Rosenhan, D. L. On being sane in insane places. *Science*, 1973, **179**, 250–258.

Ruesch, J. and Brodsky, C. M. The concept of social disability. *Archives of General Psychology*, 1968, **19**, 394–403.

Salzinger, K. Discussion of vocal measures and drug effects. In K. Salzinger and S. Salzinger (Eds.), *Research in verbal behavior and some neurophysiological implications*. New York: Academic, 1967.

Sarbin, T. R. The scientific status of the mental illness metaphor. In S. C. Plog and R. B. Edgerton (Eds.), *Changing perspectives in mental illness*. New York: Holt, Rinehart & Winston, 1969.

Schiørring, E. and Randrup, A. Social isolation and changes in the formation of groups induced by amphetamine in an open field test with rats. In O. Vinar, Z. Votava, and P. B. Bradley (Eds.), *Advances in neuropsychopharmacology*. Amsterdam: North-Holland, 1971.

Scott, J. P. The social psychology of infrahuman animals. In G. Lindzey and E. Aronson (Eds.), *The handbook of social psychology*. Vol. 4., 2nd ed. Reading, Mass.: Addison-Wesley, 1969.

Shapiro, D. and Crider, A. Psychophysiological approaches in social psychology. In G. Lindzey and E. Aronson (Eds.), *The handbook of social psychology*. Vol. 3, 2nd ed. Reading, Mass.: Addison-Wesley, 1969.

Smythies, J. R. The mode of action of psychotomimetic drugs. In F. O. Schmitt, G. Adelman, T. Melnechuk, and F. G. Worden (Eds.), *Neurosciences research symposium summaries*. Vol. 5. Cambridge, Mass.: MIT Press, 1971.

Spiegel, R. Battegay, R., and Abt, K. Comparative study of the effects produced by psychotropic drugs on verbal interaction in a group of students. In O. Vinar, Z. Votava, and P. B. Bradley (Eds.), *Advances in neuropsychopharmacology*. Amsterdam: North-Holland, 1971.

Stone, P. J., Dunphy, D. C., Smith, M. S., and Ogilvie, D. M. *The General Enquirer: A computer approach to content analysis*. Cambridge Mass.: MIT Press, 1966.

Szasz, T. S. *The myth of mental illness*. New York: Harper & Row, 1961.

Trott, D. M. and Morf, M. E. A multi-method factor analysis of the Differential Personality Inventory, Personality Research Form, and Minnesota Multiphasic Personality Inventory. *Journal of Counseling Psychology*, 1972, **19**, 94–100.

Vance, E. T. Social disability. *American Psychologist*, 1973, **28**, 498–511.

Waskow, I. E. The effects of drugs on speech: A review. In K. Salzinger, and S. Salzinger (Eds.), *Research in verbal behavior and some neurophysiological implications*. New York: Academic, 1967 *(a)*

Waskow, I. E. Vocal measures and drug effects. In K. Salzinger and S. Salzinger (Eds.), *Research in verbal behavior and some neurophysiological implications*. New York: Academic, 1967. *(b)*

Webb, E. J., Campbell, D. T., Schwartz, R. D., and Sechrest, L. *Unobtrusive measures: Nonreactive research in the social sciences*. Chicago: Rand McNally, 1966.

Weick, K. E. Systematic observational methods. In G. Lindzey and E. Aronson (Eds.), *The handbook of social psychology*. Vol. 2., 2nd ed. Reading, Mass.: Addison-Wesley, 1968.

Weiss, R. L. Operant conditioning techniques in psychological assessment. In P. McReynolds (Ed.), *Advances in psychological assessment*. Vol. 1. Palo Alto: Science and Behavior Books, 1968.

Wittenborn, J. R., Goldberg, S. C., and May, P. R. A. *Psychopharmacology and the individual patient*. New York: Raven, 1970.

Zajonc, R. B. *Animal social psychology: A reader of experimental studies*. New York: Wiley, 1969.

Zimmer, J. M. and Cowles, K. H. Content analysis using FORTRAN: Applied to interviews conducted by C. Rogers, F. Perls, and A. Ellis. *Journal of Consulting Psychology*, 1972, **19**, 161–166.

CHAPTER 3

# Social Judgment Theory:
# Its Use in the Study of Psychoactive Drugs

KENNETH R. HAMMOND


The present chapter describes social judgment theory and its application to the study of the effects of psychoactive drugs on human judgment. The principal concepts, the models, the quantitative methods, the research methods, and the set of problems encompassed by the theory are described.


## SOCIAL JUDGMENT THEORY

Social judgment theory is founded on the work of Egon Brunswik and Edward Tolman. It is, therefore, a cognitive, rather than a stimulus-response theory. As the name of the theory suggests, it is restricted to the process of human judgment, particularly as that process is applied to social, rather than physical, events. It can hardly be considered to encompass a narrow set of problems, however, inasmuch as human judgment is one of man's more important cognitive capabilities. Indeed, judgment may be man's *most* important cognitive capability. The possession of good judgment is considered to be the mark of wisdom. Good judgment is, in principle, the *sine qua non* for persons selected for positions of large responsibility. At the other extreme, the failure to be able to execute the minimum requisite amount of good judgment results in persons being labeled dangerous to themselves or society and, in consequence, being removed from society and placed under surveillance in jails or hospitals where, it is hoped, good judgment can somehow be restored.

Although the importance of human judgmental processes is never disputed, its broader aspects have only recently become the object of scientific inquiry. Therefore, little is known about this aspect of our cognitive activity. Studies of judgment were undertaken early in the history of psychology, but they involved judgments in relation to sensory and perceptual functions which, for example, compared weights or sizes of different physical objects. Results of such studies, however, have little bearing on the more complex, everyday aspects of human judgment: about other persons; regarding choice of occupation; judgments involved in the formulation or implementation of social policies, and so forth. It is only since the period after World War II that the more complex human judgments began to be studied, and only since 1960 that research has begun in earnest.

There is, of course, more than one approach to the study of human judgment. Only social judgment theory has been applied to the study of the effects of psychoactive drugs, however, and therefore, only social judgment theory will be considered here. (See, however, Slovic & Lichtenstein, 1973, for a review of various approaches.)

## Basic Premises

Social judgment theory is based on the proposition that, in social life, conclusions must be drawn with regard to cognitive tasks that are not wholly susceptible to analytical processes. As a result, it is necessary for persons to make use of what has traditionally been called "judgment." There is, for example, no analytical process, no formula, that the ordinary person can apply to cognitive tasks such as deciding where to spend a holiday, whom to trust, how to make best use of money, whether to continue one's education, or to such major policy questions as whether to extend or decrease foreign aid, whether to form an alliance with this nation or that one, and so on. All tasks of this sort are dealt with in terms of human judgment, and often the person making the judgment is under the influence of a psychoactive drug, such as alcohol. And, because judgments involve a covert, largely nonrecoverable, process, it is largely mysterious to layman and scientist alike. The layman is apt to limit his description of the process to something like "a conclusion reached on balance." Of the several definitions offered by Webster's Second International Dictionary (unabridged) two are closely related to the present usage: ". . . The mental act of judging; the operation of the mind, involving comparison and discrimination, by which knowledge of values and relations is mentally formulated; as, by a series of wrong *judgments* he forfeited confidence. . . . The power of arriving at a wise decision or conclusion on the basis of indications and probabilities, when the facts are not clearly ascertained; as, to use your best *judgment*; discretion; discernment; as, a man of sound *judgment*."

The view of the process offered by Webster may be found throughout history. And although the traditional view serves as a useful point of departure, the covert nature of the process, together with the esteem in which the practitioners of judgment are held, encourages the layman (and often scientists as well) to assume that human judgment is beyond empirical analysis. Such assumptions are no doubt partly responsible for the long delay in the application of scientific methods to its study. The purpose of the present chapter, however, is to show that a theory of human judgment can be applied to specific empirical problems, such as ascertaining the effects on human judgment of biochemical changes induced in the nervous system by psychoactive drugs. Our first step toward that goal requires that we call attention to a distinction between analytical and intuitive modes of thought, and to introduce a concept unfamiliar to most readers—quasirational cognition.

## Quasirational Cognition

The analytical process has received by far the greatest attention by students of human thought; there have been far fewer empirical attempts to cope with the form of cognition known as intuition. Even less work has been directed toward what is here (and elsewhere, see Brunswik, 1966; Hammond, 1966, 1972) called quasirational thought. As used in the context of social judgment theory, quasirational thought refers to the type of cognition involved in judgment—a synthesis of analysis and intuition, a matter we now consider in detail.

In the attempt to apply knowledge to a social task, analytical processes will be used when possible, but analytical processes cannot take one very far in coping with the cognitive tasks of everyday life. There is no set of theoretical principles or empirical rules which can ordinarily be applied to other than the most elementary of these tasks. Although a person cannot ignore analytical forms of thought without being accused of irresponsibility and capriciousness, if one persists in applying analytical forms of cognition to problems in which there is little or no justification for their use, errors of judgment are apt to be large. Paranoid schizophrenic patients are traditionally accused of inappropriate applications of analytical thought (indeed, inappropriate analytical thought tends to be a defining characteristic of paranoia), but they are not alone in this regard. Professional students of society, economists, sociologists, psychoanalysts, and psychologists as well as politicians and idealogues often make large errors of judgment because of an overly analytical and doctrinaire application of knowledge. On the other hand, an extended use of intuitive thought without attendant checks from analysis may be equally unsatisfactory. Errors resulting from inappropriate use of intuitive thought are not apt to be catastrophic, however, as errors resulting from analytical thought are apt to be (see Brunswik, 1956).

The usual mode of thought persons apply to cognitive tasks in the ordinary course of events is a quasirational mode, in which elements of *both* analysis and intuition are required. To what extent more or less of either element is applied in a given situation is generally an individual matter. For some people in some situations, analysis will be used if and when and where it can be, and intuition will be called upon to do what it can to *supplement* analysis. Other people in similar circumstances will, however, employ an intuitive mode of thought insofar as it proves useful, and employ analysis as a *check* when and if they can.

This description of the basic cognitive process upon which judgment rests is, of course, quite vague, but it will serve its purpose if it deflects the reader from the usual practice of describing thought processes in terms of rationality *or* irrationality, and if it encourages one to think, instead, in terms of a cognitive process which falls on a different dimension—namely, the analytic-intuitive dimension, and, in particular, encourages one to think of the judgment process as involving elements of both.

## Uncertainty

One of the important reasons why quasirational thought is applied to the cognitive tasks of everyday life is that *uncertainty* is embedded in such tasks. Because analytical principles cannot be applied with thoroughness, because one ordinarily does not know, and cannot know, all the factors involved in such tasks, or the nature of their relationships to one another, one must rely to some extent on *experience*. One behaves in the way one does, not only because one understands a given situation and what it requires, but also because certain behaviors have been useful in the past, irrespective of whether the situation is understood or not. Experience may provide a guide, although experience does not always reveal its source; memory is imperfect. The residues of experience are brought to bear on a given situation in ways not obvious to the person making a judgment. Moreover, as a result of the uncertainty in the cognitive tasks of everyday life, experience provides an *uncertain* guide to judgment. Uncertainty in the task and in the judgment system of the person coping with it are persistent elements of quasirational judgments.

In order to move from the foregoing vague descriptions of the judgmental process to more concrete descriptions, we turn now to a consideration of the specific concepts employed by social judgment theory and the manner in which they are linked together.

## Principal Concepts

The principal concepts of social judgment theory are best illustrated by reference to the model of the judgment situation presented in Figure 3.1. The most general

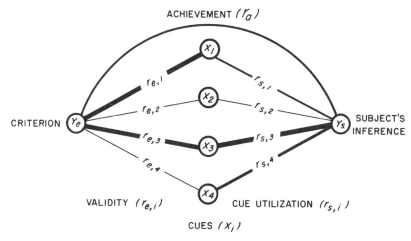

ACHIEVEMENT $(r_a)$

CRITERION $Y_e$

SUBJECT'S INFERENCE $Y_s$

VALIDITY $(r_{e,i})$

CUE UTILIZATION $(r_{s,i})$

CUES $(X_i)$

**Figure 3.1.**   A double-system judgment task showing differential weighting with respect to both the ecological validities and the cue utilizations. (Width of line indicates weight.)

proposition to be gained from Figure 3.1 is that judgment is a cognitive process similar to inductive inference, in which the person draws a conclusion, or an inference $Y_s$, about something $Y_e$, which he *cannot* see (or otherwise directly perceive), on the basis of data $X_i$, which he *can* see (or otherwise directly perceive). In other words, judgments are made from palpable data, which serve as cues to impalpable events and circumstances. The wide-ranging arc connecting $Y_s$ and $Y_e$ (labeled $r_a$ in Figure 3.1) indicates the degree to which the judgment $Y_s$ was correct; that is, the extent to which the judgment coincides with the actual circumstance to be judged. A rough example can be found in the judgments of the weather forecaster (amateur or professional) who looks at certain palpable cues $X_i$ such as wind speed, temperature, barometric pressure and makes a judgment $Y_s$ about what tomorrow's weather $Y_e$ will be. The arc $r_a$ indicates his success as a forecaster over a series of judgments.

Throughout any ordinary day one frequently encounters similar circumstances. Palpable data (e.g., events in the news, actions of friends and enemies, activities of the stock market) evoke judgments as to the unperceived events that gave rise to the events perceived. *Causes* $Y_e$ are frequently being inferred $Y_s$ from those cue-events $X_i$, or *effects,* observed. And the ability to make correct inferences (indicated by $r_a$) is, of course, an ability in which persons are believed to differ widely. High values of judgmental accuracy $r_a$ are considered to be essential attributes of persons with high responsibility; low values indicate the situation of a person very likely to be in difficulty with his social or physical surroundings.

The effects of various psychoactive drugs on judgmental accuracy have never been ascertained, although judgmental accuracy is important and such drugs are used very widely.

## Differential Weight

The model in Figure 3.1 also indicates the concept of differential weight. Cues may have differential *weight* in that they are of differential value in making inferences about events. That is, if a cue has a very strong relation (has a high degree of covariation) with an event to be inferred, it will be more useful than one which has a weak relation. Therefore cues with high degrees of covariation with the event to be inferred have a large degree of ecological validity, their weight is greater than those with low degrees of covariation.

The counterpart to the ecological validity $r_e$ of a cue is its utilization $r_s$ by the subject (see Figure 3.1). Cues also may be used or depended upon to a larger or smaller degree and, therefore, with regard to their *subjective utilization*. Thus, an observer may compare the differential weights of a set of cues $r_{ei}$ in the task with the weights implicitly assigned to them $r_{si}$ by the person making the inference. Mismatches between ecological validities and subjective utilization of cues is one source of inaccurate judgments. In other words, one source of poor judgment lies in the failure to attach the correct relative weights or importance to cues; one "balances" the information incorrectly.

As will be shown below, psychoactive drugs may enhance or impair a person's ability to weigh information correctly, and as a result, his judgmental accuracy may be enhanced or impaired accordingly.

## Function Form

Cues not only have different task weights, but they may be related to the variable to be inferred $Y_e$ by means of different functional relations, or *function forms*. These may include positive linear function forms, negative linear function forms, or a variety of curvilinear function forms (see Figure 3.2). Of course, cues may be related to judgments $Y_s$ by means of various function forms also, and the comparison, or match, between task function form and subjective function form will also provide information about the reason for accurate or inaccurate judgments.

Tasks that involve curvilinear functions are apt to be more difficult to learn than those with positive linear function forms, and people whose judgments are related

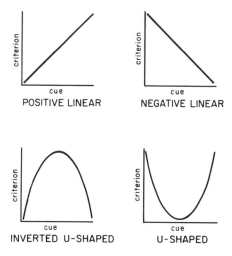

**Figure 3.2.**  Examples of linear and curvilinear function forms.

to cues in curvilinear forms are apt to be more difficult for other people to understand. Moreover, people seldom make explicit to others exactly which function form they are employing in a given situation, simply because most people are not aware of this concept. It may appear in colloquial form, however. For example, one way to indicate that another person is using a positive linear function form when he should be using a curvilinear one is to say that his error lies in believing that "if a little is good, more is better"—a rule which, if followed in the taking of medicine, is apt to lead to disaster. The reader will find it easy to think of other examples of an inappropriate use of linear function forms. One should also consider the difficulties of *changing* a function form to fit the function form of a task, or to fit one preferred by a friend, a teacher, or therapist.

As shown later, empirical analyses of the effects of psychoactive drugs on this problem are possible and informative.

### Organizing Principles

The principles by which the cue data are organized into a judgment are of considerable importance. Such data may be organized by adding them: $Y_s = X_1 + X_2 + X_3$; by averaging them: $Y_s = (X_1 + X_2 + X_3)/3$; or by making use of some configural or patterning principle: $Y_s = X_1 + X_2X_3$.

When asked about how they organize information into a judgment, most persons are apt to report that they make use of a pattern or configuration of the data. Physicians who make a diagnosis, stock market experts, and others whose professional judgment is critical generally reply to questions about their judgment processes by referring more or less vaguely to their intuitive ability to recognize "patterns." Empirical research, however, in general has not supported these contentions; simpler organizing principles have been found to account for, or at least to predict, judgments from data better than patterns. Although it hardly seems doubtful that human beings organize data by means of patterns, the extent to which they do in fact so organize data is unknown; in any event, reports of the use of such principles certainly cannot be taken for granted. To what extent psychoactive drugs affect the ability of persons to organize data into a judgment in different ways is unknown; in the studies described in this book this problem could be addressed only indirectly.

## Consistency

Finally, it is important to consider the *consistency* with which the same judgment is made in response to the same data. Although everyone is apt to assume that they always make the same judgments when confronted with the same facts, it is virtually certain that they will not do so except under the very simplest circumstances. That is, perfect consistency in judgments is apt to occur only when there is no uncertainty whatever in the task situation. Such simple task situations, of course, require little in the way of judgment, inasmuch as a given cue always evokes the same judgment.

Some diseases are of this variety, that is, they provide single cues (i.e., the same disease always produces the same symptoms), but social circumstances very seldom provide tasks of no uncertainty whatever, and to which persons can respond with perfect consistency. To what extent psychoactive drugs affect the consistency with which judgments are made is one of the questions directly investigated in this volume.

The four basic concepts described above do not exhaust the conceptual framework of social judgment theory, but they will be sufficient to describe the present empirical work undertaken to determine the effects of psychoactive drugs on human judgment. Before proceeding to the quantification of these concepts, we turn to a description of the four circumstances in which the concepts described above can be used. (For a more detailed discussion of social judgment theory, the reader may consult Hammond, Stewart, Brehmer & Steinmann, 1975.)

# EXPANSION OF THE MODEL: FOUR CASES

## Single-System Case

In this case (illustrated in Figure 3.3) the problem for the judgment theorist is to externalize, that is, to make explicit the judgmental *policy* that a person uses in connection with a specific judgment situation. For example, suppose that the task for the judgment theorist were to externalize the judgmental policy of a person who is about to purchase a car. And suppose further that there were only four aspects of an automobile that he took into consideration: its cost, its aesthetic quality, its reliability, and its horsepower. The task for the judgment theorist would be to discover (1) the relative *weight* the person assigned to each of the four cues, (2) the *function form* of each cue in relation to the person's judgment, (3) the principle by which the data from the four cues were *organized,* and (4) the *consistency* with which the judgment was exercised.

The judgment theorist might well undertake this task by presenting the person with information about a number of hypothetical cars with regard to these four characteristics, and by asking the person to exercise his preferences. The theorist then extracts, by statistical analysis, descriptions of the person's judgment policy with regard to the four parameters indicated above.

This procedure was used in the studies by Gillis (Chapter 14) in the following way. He asked patients to make judgments about the ability of a number of hypothetical psychiatrists, each of which was described in terms of three cues:

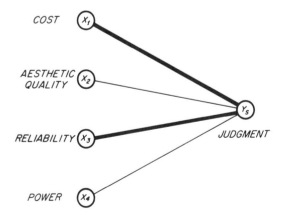

**Figure 3.3.**   A single-system judgment task.

their age, intelligence, and warmth. After the patients made their judgments on a scale from 1 to 20 with regard to "how good do you think this doctor would be," Gillis analyzed the weights and function forms used by each patient in making their judgments, as well as examining the organizing principle used, and the consistency with which the patients made their judgments. As a result, he could provide a description of each patient's judgment policy and thus compare patients with one another with regard to the four parameters described above.

It should be noted that there is no criterion available in the single-system case. That is, there is no "right answer" with which a person's judgment may be compared. The aim of studies within the single-system case, therefore, is not to determine judgmental accuracy, but simply to describe the values of the parameters of a person's judgmental system. An example of the use to which information of this sort can be put in the study of the effects of psychoactive drugs on behavior may be found in Chapter 13.

## Double-System Case

In this case (illustrated in Figure 3.1) the task includes a criterion; that is, there is some known, or soon-to-be-known, condition or variable $Y_e$, the values of which the person is trying to infer from the values of a set of cues. Because the criterion values will be known, it is thus possible to measure the *accuracy* of a person's judgment—something not possible in the single-system case. Accuracy $r_a$ is measured by comparing the judgments $Y_s$ made with the criterion values $Y_e$. Thus, in the double-system case it is possible to analyze a person's ability to learn to make correct judgments under a variety of circumstances, provided some form of feedback is offered to the learner.

Task conditions and/or subject conditions may be changed in this case and the effects of such changes on judgmental accuracy may be ascertained. For example, the effect may be examined of increasing the number of cues on the rate of learning to make correct inferences. Or, as shown in the empirical studies to follow, the effects of antipsychotic, or other psychoactive drugs, on subjects' ability to learn to make correct judgments may be ascertained.

As indicated above, the process of learning to improve one's judgments can be analyzed in terms of matches between task-system-parameter values and judgment-system-parameter values, as for example, weight, function form, or organizational principles.

# Triple-System Case

In this case (illustrated in Figure 3.4) the interaction of *two* subjects coping with a judgment task is the focus of the investigation. Typical problems of interest in the triple-system case are interpersonal conflict (involving different judgments) and interpersonal learning (involving each person's ability to learn *from* and/or *about* the other person). As in the double-system case, either task or subject conditions may be varied. Thus, the complexity of the judgment task may be varied, or, as shown in the studies reported in Part II of this volume, the effects of various psychoactive drugs on interpersonal conflict and/or interpersonal learning may be investigated.

The specific values of the parameters of the judgment systems of two persons may be compared in this case, exactly as the parameter values of a task system and a person's judgment system were compared in the double-system case. Thus, the reasons for disagreement in judgments between two persons may be traced to different parameter values being applied to the common task (see Figure 3.4). Moreover, the difference between the parameter values of two persons' judgment systems will indicate what each person has to learn *about* the other.

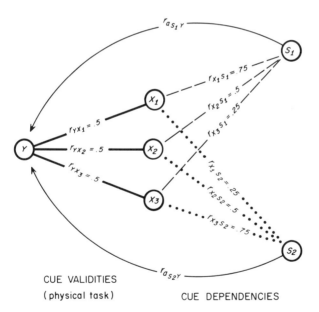

CUE VALIDITIES
(physical task)    CUE DEPENDENCIES

**Figure 3.4.**   A triple-system judgment task showing differential cue weightings of each subject and cue validities of the conflict task.

In order to determine what one person has to learn *from* the other, it is necessary to take into consideration the difference between the learner's judgment system and the task system, as well as the difference between the judgment systems of the two persons.

In short, the cognitive dynamics of both interpersonal conflict and interpersonal learning are studied within the framework of the triple-system case. Obviously, the matter is complex. However, it is precisely these circumstances that must be dealt with if we are to ascertain directly the effects of psychoactive drugs in important social situations, particularly those directed toward the improvement of cognitive functioning.

## N-System Case

In this case the number of tasks or persons is expanded to the size desired by the investigator. Since none of the studies in Part III falls within the $N$-system case, no further discussion of it is provided here (however, see Kessel, 1973; Moscovici, Lage, & Naffrechaux, 1973; Cvetkovich, 1973).

## QUANTITATIVE PROCEDURES

The concepts and models generated by social judgment theory are very well suited to analysis by means of *multiple regression* techniques; a modified form of these procedures is used to analyze the behavior of subjects in all of the four cases described above.

In its most general form, the basic proposition from which quantification follows is:

performance $= f$ (knowledge, task control, subject control)

The general statement is interpreted in this way: variations in a person's judgmental accuracy (his performance) are a function of the extent to which he has correct *knowledge* of the judgmental task, there is *task control,* and there is *judgmental control.*

*Knowledge* defines the extent to which the parameters of a person's judgmental system match those of the task system.

*Task control* defines the extent to which the variable $Y_e$ may be predicted from the cue variables $X_i$. Should the criterion variable to be inferred $Y_e$ be perfectly predictable from the cue variables $X_i$, then perfect task control exists. Task control diminishes to the extent that such predictability diminishes. Of course, task control is the inverse of uncertainty. The more uncertainty in the task system, the less task control in the task system.

*Judgmental control* includes similar reasoning. If a person's judgment $Y_s$ is perfectly predictable from the cue values $X_i$, perfect judgmental control exists. To the extent that such predictability diminishes, judgmental control diminishes. And the more uncertainty in a person's judgmental system, the less judgmental control.

The verbal form of the equation above is intended to convey the general theory upon which quantification is based, and to indicate that judgmental performance is dependent upon three main parameters. It should be noted that: *(a)* one of these (task control) is *wholly beyond* the subject's control; and *(b)* that another (knowledge) is a product of (at least) information about the task and the subject's cognitive ability, and is therefore only *partly* under the subject's control; and *(c)* that only the third parameter (judgmental control) can be said to be *wholly under* the subject's control.

The general quantitative expression of the above proposition is:

$$r_a = G\,R_e\,R_s \tag{1}$$

where   $r_a$ = achievement, or judgmental accuracy; it is equal to the correlation between $Y_s$ and $Y_e$,

$G$ = the correlation between $Y_e$ and $Y_s$, after each has been corrected for inconsistency (measured by $R_e$ and $R_s$),

$R_e$ = the consistency of the judgmental task system; it is equal to the multiple correlation between the cue values $X_i$ and the values of $Y_e$,

$R_s$ = the consistency of the person making the judgments; it is equal to the multiple correlation between the cue values $X_i$ and the values of $Y_s$.

Equation 1 has been the subject of several theoretical and quantitative analyses (see, for example, Hursch, Hammond, & Hursch, 1964; Tucker, 1964; Goldberg, 1970; Hammond & Summers, 1972; Brehmer, 1969, 1973; Stewart, 1973). It has been used to generate various quantitative measures for the analysis of judgment in each of the three cases described above. For example, as pointed out in the discussion of the verbal form of the equation, and as indicated in its mathematical form, performance or judgmental accuracy $r_a$ can be affected by three independent factors: $G$ (knowledge), $R_e$ (task control) and $R_s$ (judgmental control). Therefore, the important question that should be immediately raised about a new (or even a "well-known") drug is: does it affect judgmental performance $r_a$? If so, does it affect judgmental performance because it affects the person's ability to *acquire knowledge* of the judgmental task $G$, or his ability to *control* his judgmental processes $R_s$? In other words, does it affect his ability to acquire knowledge, or to apply it?

It is precisely such questions that are addressed by the empirical studies in Part II.

## MAJOR RESEARCH PROBLEMS

Social judgment theory has addressed itself to three major problems: (1) learning to improve judgment, (2) interpersonal conflict, and (3) interpersonal learning. Methods by which the theory and its associated quantitative procedures are applied to each of these problems follow.

### Learning to Improve Judgment

Despite the obvious importance of this process, it is only recently that psychologists have turned their attention to it; human judgment has never received any systematic study in connection with the serious degradation of cognitive functioning, or therapeutic efforts to restore it. If there is truth in the general proposition set forth earlier, namely, *(a)* that human judgment is a cognitive process which serves critical functions in everyday life, and *(b)* that the impairment of this function is apt to lead to serious difficulties including either imprisonment or hospitalization, then *(c)* surely the improvement of that process should come under *direct* scientific scrutiny. In particular, the effects of psychoactive drugs on the ability to learn to improve one's judgment should be directly examined.

The first three studies in Part II examine the problem of judgmental learning. The general method and procedures involved are discussed below.

#### Method and Procedure

The study of judgmental learning falls within the double-system case. A judgment task is constructed so that it includes the parameters the investigator considers to be appropriate to a given study. Thus, for example, a task may be constructed so that (as in Figure 3.1) it includes three cues $X_i$ each with a specified relation $r_e$ to the criterion $Y_e$, and with a specified function form (positive or negative linear or curvilinear), with a specified degree of uncertainty $R_e$, and with a specified organizational principle (an additive, averaging, or configural, "patterning" principle). The cues are typically represented by bar graphs as in Figure 3.5, in which the cue values are represented by the height of the bars. The correct (criterion) values are also represented numerically.

The subject may observe the value of the three cues by observing the height of three bars, and, upon being requested to do so, makes a judgment about the value of the criterion variable on the basis of the values of the three cues. The subject may then, for example, be told the correct value of the criterion variable (that is, be told the judgment that should have been made). The subject is then shown a second set of cue values, asked to make a judgment, then shown the correct judgment, and so on for as many trials as is appropriate for a given study.

In order to improve one's judgments, that is, in order to make one's judgments approximate (or covary with) the correct answer, the learner should, in general, adjust subjective weights to approximate those of the task, and similarly adjust function forms to match the task-function forms, and to use the appropriate way of organizing the cue data into a judgment with a high degree of consistency. The investigator may thus observe not only the *rate* at which the learner's judgment improves, but also the *manner* in which the learner improves it. That is, the investigator may observe whether the subject proceeds by adjusting weights, *or* by adjusting function forms, and how the subject organized the data into a judgment. The investigator may also observe whether achievement is limited by a failure to *acquire* the correct knowledge of the judgment task, or through a failure to *apply* effectively the knowledge he acquired. Each of these concepts is discussed in turn.

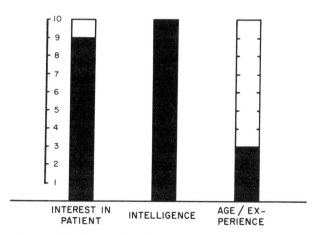

**Figure 3.5.**  An example of cue information in bar-graph form.

*Performance*.   The subject's over-all performance is indicated by the correlation $r_a$ between his judgment and the correct value of the criterion variable. One of the first questions directed at the effects of any psychoactive drug would, of course, concern its effect on $r_a$. Several of the studies reported in Part II show that different drugs do affect the rate of growth of $r_a$, and one study shows that a widely used antipsychotic drug affects performance *adversely* in relation to a placebo in hospitalized psychotic patients. The specific conclusion drawn from these results is that the ability of such patients to learn to improve their judgment is impaired by the drug in question. Because the parameters of judgmental task systems are representative of the parameters of such tasks in social life, the general conclusion drawn from this result is that the ability of patients to improve their judgment in social life outside the specific task situation may well be impaired by the drug in question. At the very least, such results indicate that the person who administers the drug should consider the possible "social toxicity" of the drug.

*Knowledge*.   As indicated, the reasons for the patient's failure or enhanced ability to improve performance $r_a$ adequately under administration of a specific drug might be due to the effect of the drug on the patient's ability to acquire correct knowledge of specific task parameters. This ability is reflected by the measure $G$ in (1). Acquisition of knowledge about the task may also be analyzed in more specific terms by comparing subjective cue utilization $r_s$ with objective weights $r_e$, and by comparing function forms used by the subjects with task function forms, and so forth.

In several of the studies described in Part II, specific comparisons were made between $r_s$ (the subjects' dependence on, or utilization of, a cue) and $r_e$ (the weight or validity of that cue in a judgment task). Moreover, analyses were made of the ability of a subject who had received various drugs to learn to place appropriate weight on a cue with a curvilinear rather than a linear function form. Thus, the ability to acquire the knowledge necessary to improve judgment was analyzed in terms of the specific parameters of that process.

*Control*.   Several previous studies of learning to improve judgment suggest that acquisition of knowledge precedes the ability to control its application successfully (Hammond & Summers, 1972). As (1) indicates, performance would be enhanced or impaired if a psychoactive drug acts to change the value of $R_s$; that is, performance would be enhanced or impaired insofar as a person's control over the execution or application of knowledge already acquired is affected by a drug. As illustrated in the studies in Part II, $R_s$ is a useful parameter of the judgment process; it provides a measure of cognitive control that is sensitive to psychoactive drugs.

*Feedback.*    The concept of feedback occupies a special place in the study of human judgment and will be given special consideration here. As mentioned, in the past, studies of human judgment were considered to be somewhat unconventional from the learning psychologist's point of view and indeed, there has been a tendency to disparage studies of judgmental learning because they have little in common with the traditional study of judgment or learning. Unfortunately, as it turns out, until about 1970, studies of judgmental learning had *too much* in common with traditional ways of studying learning. The concept in common was that of *outcome feedback.*

Consider the typical judgmental learning study described. Recall that after each judgment is made, the learner is told the correct answer; that is, he is given the outcome for the trial. Such outcome feedback, as in conventional studies of learning, was provided in order for the learner to learn; without receiving such outcome feedback, without receiving the correct answer on each trial, there would be little reason to expect learning to occur. So, without giving the matter much thought, psychologists studying judgmental learning routinely provided outcome feedback for their subjects. Under these conditions, learning was slow, boring, and "stupid," in the sense that subjects were poor at reporting what they had learned. (For a review, see Slovic & Lichtenstein, 1973.)

Only after some years of research did it become apparent that studies of judgmental learning were providing their subjects with tasks that not only were very difficult, but also were of doubtful meaning, precisely because of a thoughtless adherence to a concept ingrained in traditional learning theory—information through outcomes. However useful the observations of outcomes might be in traditional learning tasks, outcome feedback offers very little helpful information if a task contains a number of cues, and if those cues have different weights and different function forms, and if there is uncertainty in the relations between cue and criterion. Indeed, if outcomes are the only feedback provided, then learning will require hundreds if not thousands of trials, and tasks with nonlinear function forms will be particularly difficult if not impossible to learn (Deane, Hammond, & Summers, 1972). Moreover, reflection on this matter will remind the reader that in social life, outcome feedback occurs infrequently in relation to his judgments and that it is seldom helpful when it does occur. Rather, learning to improve one's judgment ordinarily occurs as a result of some person pointing out to the learner a *discrepancy* between the weight, or importance, the learner is attaching to certain cues and their actual importance in the judgment task.

Thus, for example, a mother who wishes to help her child improve the accuracy of his or her judgment of people points out that a foreign accent, or the unusual customs of a foreigner, are not good cues to intelligence, or other personal characteristics. And should her child make judgments which the mother considers incorrect about the personal characteristics of other persons, she will point out the discrepancy between the manner in which she thinks the various cues ought to be weighted and the manner in which she thinks the child is weighting them. The same holds true for other parameters of judgmental systems, insofar as the mother, or teacher, is aware of them. This form of feedback, which is directed toward the relation between the parameters of judgment tasks and judgment systems, is called *cognitive feedback,* in contrast to *outcome feedback* (see Hammond & Brehmer, 1973; Hammond, 1971; Hammond & Summers, 1972).

There are two reasons for what may appear to the reader to be a digression about the concept of feedback. The first is that it is only recently that the distinction between the two forms of feedback has become apparent, and the reader may not be familiar with it. The second reason is that the distinction has important consequences for the study of psychoactive drugs on learning to improve judgment. Because of the recency of the introduction of the concept of cognitive feedback, and because of the technical problems in providing it in a form readily grasped by patients, few studies of the effects of psychoactive drugs on learning to improve judgment have provided cognitive feedback for learners. (See, however, Chapters 14 and 15 of this volume.)

## Interpersonal Conflict

A second major research problem, the study of interpersonal conflict, falls within the triple-system case. The three systems include a single-task system and two-person systems. Before presenting the details of the method and procedure used in the study of interpersonal conflict (IPC), it will be useful to consider the problem of IPC from the point of view of social judgment theory, inasmuch as social judgment theory treats IPC in a nonconventional way.

The conventional view of interpersonal conflict argues that the cause of conflict is differential personal gain—in a word, greed. Because of psychology's long history of involvement with the study of motivation (including the enormous emphasis given to the topic by Freud) virtually all psychological explanations of conflict are motivational explanations. It is generally assumed, for example, that motives distort cognitive and perceptual functions to the point where persons behave irrationally. As a result of roughly 75 years of work, the basic conclusion of the twentieth century is that only *rational men of good will* can successfully settle their differences—other than by accident. Unhappily, this conclusion is tempered by a corollary, namely that the ubiquitousness of self-serving motives makes good will, and therefore rationality, a rare event. Consequently, conflict is to be expected until self-serving motives are somehow reduced or eliminated. Implicit in this widely held point of view is the assumption that if man's reason were not distorted by his motives, his cognitive powers *would* enable him to settle his differences in a rational way. In short, man's *unlimited* cognitive powers are *flawed* by his motives.

Social judgment theory has an alternative view; it argues that man's cognitive powers are not *flawed*, rather, they are *limited*. Without denying the fact that quarrels often do arise in circumstances involving differential gain, social judgment theory argues that perhaps the largest number of quarrels arise in circumstances in which differential gain is not involved, but where a high degree of mutual interest is involved. Indeed, aside from quarrels over "who gets what" (differential gain) there are a number of types of quarrels that are highly cognitive in origin, and which are seldom considered when interpersonal conflict is discussed. There are, for example, quarrels over values ("what ought to be"), over predictions ("what will be"), over methods ("how to cope"), as well as over achievements ("what has been"), all of which have their origin in cognitive functions, and all of which have largely been ignored in the study of human conflict in the enthusiasm for reducing all quarrels to those of a motivational character (see Hammond & Boyle, 1971).

The bland indifference of students of behavior to conflicts that arise from cognitive differences between persons has had particularly unfortunate consequences for those whose judgment is deemed to be so poor that they are removed from society. Because of the quick resort to motivational explanations of poor judgment, particularly by psychotherapists of virtually all persuasions, interpersonal conflicts are immediately attributed to motivational distortions of reason. The problem, then, for the therapist is to discover and to reveal the motivational origins of the impairment of cognitive functions. Explanations that deal directly with cognitive factors are seldom offered, however, primarily because there has been so little research in the field of cognition in general, and judgment in particular, that there are few cognitive explanations available to compete with motivational explanations.

Social judgment theory, however, argues that every person's cognitive functions are limited; no appeal needs to be made to the distorting effects of motives (or personality) in order to explain defective judgments. If a person's social judgment functions are defective in interpersonal situations, then efforts should be made to study and thus to understand the nature of cognitive functions in such situations. Appeals to noncognitive functions are legitimate, of course, but some prior effort should be made to understand the cognitive requirements of the tasks.

This argument applies with particular force to persons diagnosed and hospitalized as schizophrenic. Not only is their judgment deemed to be poor in the double-system case, it is notoriously bad in circumstances where their judgments conflict with those made by others (i.e., in the triple-system case). Rather than look for motivational explanations for these cognitive difficulties, social judgment theory focuses on the cognitive requirements of situations which evoke conflicting judgments; it then analyzes the cognitive processes brought to bear on them. The general theory and quantitative method used for this purpose have been described; we turn now to specific research procedures used in the study of interpersonal conflict.

### Method and Procedure

As Figure 3.4 illustrates, (1) can be applied directly to the triple-system case. The general basis of social judgment theory can, therefore, be applied to the relation between *two* sets of judgments and a task system, as well as to the relation between one set of judgments and a set of task data. These relations can be analyzed in terms of the theory and quantitative procedures employed in the double-system case. An example of how theory and quantitative method generalize from the double-system case to the triple-system case is given in Chapters 4 and 7.

We turn now to the procedures for studying cognitive conflict between persons.

### Description of the Research Paradigm

*Requirements.* The paradigm should possess sufficient rigor to allow clear denotation and quantitative specification of both task and cognitive parameters; results should meet customary scientific criteria so that research psychologists can use the paradigm in their scientific work on the problem. At the same time, however, the behavior of the subjects must possess sufficient richness and complexity so that the results of the research can be brought to bear on the problems it was intended to cope with. Not only should the paradigm provide appropriate scientific data, but also researchers from various disciplines should find the research conditions to be reasonable; the implications of the results should be direct and obvious. The paradigm described below provides the phenomena we think the investigator should see, makes it possible for him to learn what we think he should learn, meets the criteria of scientific respectability, and provides results that can be readily communicated to investigators with different backgrounds.

*Situation.* The research paradigm produces the following situation: two persons who (1) attempt to solve problems that concern both of them; (2) have mutual utilities (their gain or loss derives from their approximations to the solution of the problem); (3) receive different training in the solution of a problem involving uncertain inference. They are then brought together and find themselves dealing with a familiar problem which their experience apparently prepared them for, but (4) find that their answers differ, and that neither answer is as good as it has been, although each answer is defensible. And (5) they provide a joint decision as to the correct solution, and therefore (6) must adapt to one another as well as to the task if they are to solve their problems.

The method involves two stages: *(a)* a *learning* stage in which two subjects are trained in such a way that each learns to think differently about a common set of problems, and *(b)* a *conflict* stage in which the two subjects are brought together and attempt to arrive at joint decisions concerning the problems. The learning and conflict phases are discussed in turn.

*Learning (Training) Stage.* The aim of the learning stage is to develop different sets of cue dependencies in two subjects. For example, in a three-cue probability task, Subject #1 will learn to depend heavily on Cue $X_1$, less heavily on Cue $X_2$, and least on Cue $X_3$. Subject #2 will learn the reverse system—to depend most heavily on Cue $X_3$, less on Cue $X_2$, and least on Cue $X_1$. Cognitive differences are thus "built up" in the two subjects in their separate and different learning experiences (see Figure 3.4).

Two points about this procedure should be emphasized: (1) the method is *general*, learning may be arranged to develop in subjects whatever degree and kind of cognitive differences the investigator considers appropriate; and (2) the method is *quantitative* in nature, differences in learning may be precisely specified in terms of statistical properties of the multiple cue task, and differences in cue dependencies between subjects may be precisely denoted in terms of the statistical properties of the subject's response system. The paradigm, in short, brings cognitive differences between persons under experimental control.

*Training versus "Policy Capturing."* The learning, or training, stage of the research paradigm is an extremely important aspect of the procedure. Its purpose, of course, is to establish the cognitive conditions of the study as precisely as possible; training the subjects makes it possible for the investigator to know the nature and extent of the cognitive differences between each subject, and thus to know how much conflict can be expected on each trial, and how much and what each subject has to learn from and about the other person. Therefore training has a critical role in the study of both interpersonal conflict and interpersonal learning. But the training is time consuming and of little interest to the subject. In those hospital circumstances where patients are resentful of research procedures, or where the investigator is dealing with patients who are highly distracted and distractable, the training stage may be a distinct liability to the research effort. In such cases it is possible to use a procedure known to judgment theorists as "policy capturing." The aim of policy capturing is to discover the parameter values of a person's judgmental system that are *socially* induced (rather than induced by the training stage of the research paradigm). Thus, for example, the investigator hopes to find pairs of persons whose socially induced judgmental systems are opposite (or at least different) in various parameter values, so that persons with different judgment systems can be paired—just as if their cognitive systems had been trained to be different by the investigator.

Various studies of cognitive conflict have been conducted with socially induced rather than laboratory-induced differences between subjects. The first of these (see especially Rappoport, 1969) were conducted with the aim of determining whether the training stage of the research paradigm introduced an artifact. Several studies based on "capturing" socially induced judgmental policies showed that there were no differences in results between experiments with persons whose cognitive differences were socially induced and those whose cognitive differences were laboratory induced. The training stage of the study, in short, did not produce artifactual results.

*Conflict Stage.*   At the completion of learning the subjects are told that they have mastered the learning task and that their next problem will be to apply what they have learned; furthermore, they will carry out the second part of the task with another subject.

The subjects are then asked to proceed in this way: on each trial they are to observe the data presented on the given trial, form a conclusion as to the correct answer, write down their judgment, and report this judgment to the other person. They are then to discuss whatever differences appear in order to reach a joint decision with the other person. Next they are asked to reconsider their individual decisions in light of the discussion and write down a second private decision, which remains private. At this point they are informed of the correct answer.

*Conflict Task.*   The nature of the different learning tasks determines the degree and kind of cognitive differences the two persons bring to the conflict situation, and the nature of the conflict task influences the manner in which these differences will be resolved. Thus, for example, in one training task Subject #1's cue dependencies were Cue $X_1 = .75$, Cue $X_2 = .50$, Cue $X_3 = .25$ and the cue weightings were reversed for Subject #2. In the accompanying conflict task the cue weights were set *midway* between those of each subject, Cue $X_1 = .5$, Cue $X_2$

$= .5$, Cue $X_3 = .5$. In this case, resolution of conflict in terms of compromise was therefore enhanced. Because the "truth" was nearly always somewhere between each person's judgment, a compromise decision was reached more rapidly than would otherwise have been the case.

Note again that the method is *general*; these specific conditions need not always be employed. Just as learning may be arranged to develop whatever form of cognitive differences the investigator wishes to study, conflict-task properties may be arranged to develop whatever class of phenomena the investigator wishes to study. If, for example, the investigator wished to compare the effect of *social pressure* versus *correctness* in the conflict task, conflict-task properties could be arranged to favor the cue dependencies of the person able to exert least social pressure. One could thus compare the relative weight of social pressure and "cognitive correctness."

*Basic Data Provided by the Paradigm.* The paradigm makes it possible to ascertain the following basic data:

1. $Tr_1$: The response Subject # 1 would make to the data card if he followed his training (learning) exactly.
2. $Tr_2$: Same for Subject #2.
3. $S_1$: The response $S_1$ makes to the data card and that he announces to $S_2$ (the *overt* individual judgment).
4. $S_2$: Same for Subject #2.
5. $J$: The joint decision arrived at by the two subjects.
6. $S_1'$: The *covert* response Subject # 1 makes privately after hearing Subject #2's response, hearing Subject #2's argument, and concurring in a joint decision with him.
7. $S_2'$: Same for Subject #2.
8. $Y$: The correct answer, if there were no random error in the task system.
9. $\hat{Y}$: The answer given to both subjects which includes the error in the task system; the random difference between $Y$ and $\hat{Y}$ prevents perfect solution.

These scores, presented in Figure 3.6 in diagrammatic form, provide the fundamental data of the paradigm. A brief explanation follows.

The scores $Tr_1$ and $Tr_2$ indicate the degree of underlying cognitive conflict potentially acquired by the subjects. There are major advantages in being able to specify $Tr_1$ and $Tr_2$ in a precise, quantitative way. Currently, when psychologists wish to compare reactions of persons supposed to hold different points of view, they must be satisfied with very rough approximations to the cognitive systems of

# INTRA-TRIAL EVENTS

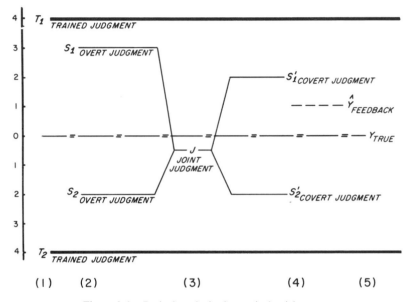

**Figure 3.6.**   Basic data obtained on a single trial.

their subjects—such approximations being obtained, for example, via "known group" techniques, or attitude-test measures. Because of the approximate nature of such data, group comparisons must be made. In contrast, $Tr_1$ and $Tr_2$ specify precisely what the differences between two specific individuals should be.

The joint decision $J$ which the subjects are required to make provides an essential element of the paradigm; it indicates the objective outcome of the discussion precipitated by the subjects' different individual judgments $S$. Subjects are required to make a second covert individual judgment $S'$ so that the effect of the negotiation over the joint decision may be ascertained. The nature of the interaction that produces $J$ may be such that the subjects harden their private $S'$ positions.

The distinction between $Y$ and $\hat{Y}$ is made mainly for technical reasons. $Y$ indicates the "answer" which would be obtained if the task involved a completely determined system. Because, as expressed earlier, the task should not be one that allows the subjects to arrive at a correct judgment on each trial in the series, $\hat{Y}$ departs randomly from $Y$. The distinction between $Y$ and $\hat{Y}$ indicates the indeterminacy in the task; the investigator may set this indeterminacy to any degree he deems appropriate to a given study.

It should be pointed out that the uncertainty in both the learning task and the conflict task provides an essential psychological component of the paradigm. In the learning stage, the investigator may arrange for his subjects to develop any degree of competence (and confidence) he believes necessary for his study by his choice of amount of uncertainty in the task. The same is true for the conflict stage. The uncertainty in the task results in the subject being uncertain whether the failure to get every answer right is due to the characteristics of the task, to his own faulty thought processes, or to the incompetence of the other person.

Various measures may readily be derived from the basic data described above; three examples follow.

1. *Compromise:* A comparison of $S$ (individual judgment) and $J$ (joint decision) provides an *overt* measure of compromise $(S - J)$; for example, if $J$ is increasingly found to be midway between $S_1$ and $S_2$ over trials, then we find increasing compromise; if $J$ is increasingly found to favor either $S_1$ or $S_2$ we find increasing capitulation. A second measure $(S' - J)$ provides an indication of compromise on a *covert* level, for neither subject reports to the other what his final $S'$ judgment is. *Overt* compromise may, of course, be affected by one set of conditions while *covert* compromise may be affected by another.

2. *Conflict:* A comparison of $Tr_1$ and $Tr_2$ indicates what the difference between the subjects' responses would be if they followed their learning exactly. The difference $(S_1 - S_2)$ is a direct measure of the overt conflict that occurs as a result of $(Tr_1 - Tr_2)$.

A second measure $(S_1' - S_2')$ indicates the *covert* conflict that remains after negotiation has taken place. It is a direct measure that may, of course, be affected by conditions different from those measuring overt conflict $(S_1 - S_2)$.

3. *Cognitive change with respect to the conflict task*: It will be remembered that the conflict task is different from the task the subjects were trained on. Thus, each subject is required to adapt to the new task by giving up, to a certain extent, his dependency on the cue he has been trained to rely on, and to develop, to a certain extent, a dependency on the cue the other person was trained to depend on. The difference $(S - Y)$ provides a measure of each subject's adaptation to the new task; the difference $(J - Y)$ provides a measure of the extent to which the subjects' joint decision approaches the correct answer in the new task.

4. *Cognitive change with respect to the other person:* Not only does the new task induce each subject to depart from his training, but also each subject induces the other to make a decision different from what his training would require. The difference $(Tr - S)$ provides a measure of the extent to which a subject's decision *overtly* departs from what his training would suggest. The difference $(Tr - S')$ provides a measure of the extent to which a subject's decision *covertly* departs

from what his training would suggest. And the difference $(S_1 - S'_1)$ indicates the extent to which a subject's *covert* decision approximates (after discussion) his previously announced decision (see Hammond, 1965).

## Implementation

In one learning task, the $Ss$ were required to learn to estimate the "level of democratic institutions" in a given nation on the basis of two cues: *(a)* the extent to which free elections existed in the nation, and *(b)* the extent to which state control was a factor in the government.

Each member of a pair of $Ss$ received different training. Subject #1 was given a task in which the "state control" variable accounted for 98% of the variance in the "level of democratic institutions" (criterion) variable. Furthermore, the "state control" variable was related to the criterion variable in a nonlinear (one phase of a sine function) manner. Thus, both low and high degrees of state control indicated a low "level of democratic institutions" and a moderate level of state control indicated a high "level of democratic institutions." For Subject #1, the second predictor variable (free elections) was *randomly* related to the criterion variable. Subject #1, then, built up a high degree of dependency on "state control" as an indicator of "level of democratic institutions."

Subject #2 learned in the opposite way; for him, "free elections" accounted for 98% of the variance in the criterion, and it was related to the criterion in a linear way. The "state control" variable, however, was *randomly* related to the criterion. Subject #2, then, built up a high degree of dependency on "free elections" as an indicator of "level of democratic institutions." (See Hammond & Summers, 1965, and Summers & Hammond, 1966, for theoretical and experimental analyses of the simultaneous learning of linear and nonlinear relationships; see also Brehmer & Hammond, 1973, for a study of the effect of different function forms on interpersonal conflict and learning.)

After each subject had reached criterion performance in training they were brought together in pairs, each member of a pair having received different training as described above. The subjects were told that they had grasped the policy in principle, and now the question was, how well could they apply it to problems involving real nations? Furthermore, "we want to see how well two of you can do the job." As indicated earlier, a data card was presented, each subject recorded an individual judgment $(S_1, S_2)$ concerning the "level of democratic institutions," each subject presented his judgment to the other and the subjects discussed their differences (cognitive differences bound to occur as a result of differential training) until they reached a joint decision $J$, then recorded a second private judgment $S'_1, S'_2$ which was not revealed to the other person; the experimenter then reported the correct answer for that task, the trial was concluded, and another begun. This general research paradigm has been employed in a number of studies since 1965. (See References, Articles on Interpersonal Conflict.) It was successfully employed by the authors of Chapters 7, 8, and 9. In the studies reported there, the quantitative method described in connection with (1) was used. Thus, agreement was measured over blocks of trials in terms of $r_a$. The components of agreement, the extent to which the two judgment policies came to match one another $G$, and the consistency, or control the subjects exercised over their judgment policies $R_s$, were also investigated.

Both types of measurement have their advantages and disadvantages, a technical matter that need not be discussed here. It is, however, worth noting that the use of (1) provides the researcher with the ability to discover whether agreement $r_a$ is lower than it should be because of a failure of judgment policies to converge (indicated by a low value of $G$), or a failure of cognitive control over judgments. Because of the suspected importance of the latter concept, the performance of subjects was measured in terms of the concepts described in (1).

### Interpersonal Conflict and Psychoactive Drugs

Previously it was argued that the effects of psychoactive drugs on learning to improve one's judgment were of such obvious importance that they deserved direct observation. Laboratory studies involving controlled quantitative analyses should be made of the behavior of the subjects attempting to improve their judgment, rather than relying on indirect methods, such as ratings (themselves badly understood judgments) made by professionals or others. The same argument applies with equal or greater cogency in connection with interpersonal conflict arising from cognitive differences. For it is the ability to cope with expressions of opinion differing from one's own in a socially acceptable way that is critical to participation in social life. Day-to-day occurrences frequently evoke conflicting judgments, most of which find no ready outcome to prove the correctness of the conflicting judgments. In any case, the vast majority of outcomes are known to be so error-ridden that credibility is always arguable. It is these circumstances that test the ability of a person to live comfortably with his fellow men and women, that test one's ability to achieve a reputation for soundness of mind. And it is the repeated failure to cope with conflicting judgments in an acceptable way that leads to suspicions of ''mental illness.'' It is important, therefore, that this ability should come under *direct* scrutiny in laboratory-controlled conditions involving quantitative analysis. When the effects of psychoactive drugs are evaluated, the research methods and procedures should combine rigorous analysis with the complexity of interpersonal conflict. For without such direct observation, the effects of such drugs on the ability to cope with interpersonal conflict can only be indirectly inferred, a procedure which, because of its indirectness, clearly requires validation. Unfortunately, validation of indirect observation has been elusive.

The research paradigm described above does provide for the rigorous, quantitative, direct examination of interpersonal conflict in complex social circumstances that are derived from a theory of human judgment. In short, it provides precisely the circumstances in which psychoactive drugs (and other factors) should be evaluated if the cognitive aspects of interpersonal conflict are to be understood.

## Interpersonal Learning

Aside from, or in addition to, the ever-recurring problem of managing interpersonal conflict, two significant questions remain: (1) what does one person learn *from* the other person as a result of the comparison of conflicting judgments, and (2) what does one person learn *about* the judgmental system of the other? Both processes are key functions in social life, and failure in either is apt to be as critical as failure in conflict management, or in learning to improve one's judgment. Indeed, learning to improve one's judgment is highly dependent upon being able to learn from another person *(a)* what the other believes the values of the judgment task parameters are, *(b)* what the values of the parameters of one's own judgmental system are, and *(c)* the discrepancy between the two. Cognitive feedback of this sort is precisely what is exchanged between persons more or less successfully in social life, as well as in the research paradigm described above.

In addition to providing an opportunity for learning about task characteristics *from* the other person, the research paradigm also provides an opportunity for each person to learn *about* the judgmental system of the other. For when Subject #1 observes Subject #2 making a judgment in response to a certain set of cue values, #1 has an opportunity to learn, for example, that #2 places a high weight on Cue $X_1$ and little weight on Cue $X_2$, and/or that #2's judgments tend to be related to Cue $X_1$ in a positive linear way, and to Cue $X_2$ in a curvilinear way.

Because the research paradigm offered the possibility of studying the effects of psychoactive drugs on interpersonal learning (IPL)—both with regard to what is learned *from* and *about* the other person—the studies included in Part II examined these processes as well as those involved in interpersonal conflict. As in the interpersonal conflict situation, the triple-system case model and (1) are directly applicable, and the same measures described there are employed in the study of IPL.

One should not lose sight of the fact that the research paradigm employed for the study of interpersonal learning involves an *interactive situation*; two (or more) persons *exchange* information about the task and themselves. One way to see the importance of this process is to compare the present research paradigm with that employed by "social learning theory" (see, for example, Bandura, 1971). For within that framework, one person is directed to learn from another person by observational means alone; there is no exchange between the person who is the subject of the study and the model (person) observed. The subject does not produce changes, nor are changes induced in the subject, by virtue of interaction with the model. Change is induced in the subject only as a result of *observation* of the model's interaction with the task situation. Thus, social learning theory is applied to a restricted, if not peculiar, set of social circumstances.

The interpersonal learning situation employed by social judgment theory, on the other hand, does in fact represent those circumstances which are critical to social learning, namely, the *exchange* of information. Failure to learn from (or about) another person in these circumstances is bound to bring risks to participation in social life. Each of these processes is discussed in turn. (See Earle, 1973, for a more detailed analysis of this point.)

### Interpersonal Learning From the Other

Conclusions may be drawn about the extent to which one person has learned from the other and the specific nature of what has been learned by analyzing the change in the parameters of the learner's judgmental policy. For example, suppose that two persons are making judgments with regard to a cognitive task involving two cues (Cue $X_1$ and Cue $X_2$). Suppose further that Subject #1 brings to the task situation a policy which includes a very high weight on Cue $X_1$ and a very low weight on Cue $X_2$, and that Subject #2 brings a judgmental policy which is exactly the opposite (a high weight on Cue $X_2$ and a low weight on Cue $X_1$). By examining the changes in cue weights, the investigator may observe whether #1 is learning from #2, #2 is learning from #1, or whether both learn from one another. For if #1 decreases the weight placed on Cue $X_1$, and increases the weight placed on Cue $X_2$, #1 is learning a new judgmental policy from #2. On the other hand, if #2 increases the weight placed on Cue $X_1$, #2 is learning from #1. (The influence of information from the task can be ignored at this point but, of course, *task* information as well as information from #2 could lead to changes in #1's policy; Hammond, 1972. Brehmer, 1973, has carried out several studies with regard to task and person effects.)

The question of the extent to which #1 has learned from #2 can be measured in terms of the change in any specific judgment parameter, such as cue weights, for example. The question of what is learned from the other may also be evaluated in terms of the *number of parameters* of the judgmental policy that were changed as a result of the interaction between #1 and #2. Thus, in the example above, #1 may have learned not only to change #1's cue-weighting system, but also to change the function form by which Cue $X_1$ was related to #1's judgment. Subject #1's judgment may have been made as a positive linear function of Cue $X_1$ prior to the interaction with #2, and then he may have learned from #2 to make judgments from Cue $X_1$ in a curvilinear manner. Or, #1 might have learned from #2 to organize the data from the task in a configural, patterned way instead of an additive manner (see Brehmer & Hammond, 1973).

In short, the research paradigm derived from the principal concepts of social judgment theory encourages the study of interpersonal learning in complex circumstances; it permits the analysis of how much and what one person learns from another in circumstances where information is exchanged. It is particularly important to note that, as in social life, the research paradigm requires that one person must learn from another while *changing* the other, and while *being changed* by the other. Such learning is difficult, involving as it does the vagaries of quasirational cognition and the dynamics of interaction. Difficult as this process might be for human beings to cope with, and difficult as it might be for psychologists to reproduce and to analyze, this is the cognitive basis of personal interaction. Therefore, we must do what we can to understand it, and to understand how psychoactive drugs affect it. A first step in this direction was undertaken in the present work; it is described in Chapters 10, 11, 12, and 13.

Studies which investigate the effects of psychoactive drugs should not only teach us about the differential sensitivity of various parameters of the interpersonal learning process to various drugs, they should also enable us to discriminate more effectively between those drugs which impair and those which enhance the ability to learn from another person. Indeed, enhancement of this process in normal persons may turn out to be as important as preventing its impairment in others.

## Interpersonal Learning About the Other

A second aspect of the interpersonal exchange of judgments concerns the nature of what the two (or more) persons learn *about* one another. This sort of learning is ordinarily epiphenomenal; that is, persons are seldom *directed* to learn about one another. Learning about the other is generally, although by no means always, incidental to the circumstances in which differing judgments are produced.

When judgments differ, however, persons will be more or less sensitive to the nature of the other's judgment policy which produced the different judgment. Clearly, the quality of the interchange between the persons will be enhanced if each person can discern correctly the characteristics of the policy of the other. If two persons can, in fact, learn about one another's judgmental policy, they will be able to predict accurately the specific judgments the other will make in response to certain cues. Such predictive accuracy is obviously of benefit in a number of ways. One of its benefits is that it enables each person to guide his behavior appropriately in relation to the other. Failure to understand the other, and thus to be unable to predict his judgments, will, of course, lead to a variety of difficulties in social interactions.

As in learning from another, one person ordinarily learns about another in circumstances of mutual exchange. That is, learning about the other frequently, if not always, takes place while learning from the other or while teaching the other. As indicated, interpersonal learning is embedded in a complex social situation which the research paradigm (employed to study the effects of psychoactive drugs) should attempt to represent. The technical difficulties of representing such circumstances, as well as the pre-eminence of theoretical orientations that tend to ignore the need for such representativeness, however, have resulted in the failure of psychologists to study seriously either form of interpersonal learning discussed here. Consequently, despite the obvious importance of both, almost nothing is known about either process.

The analysis of the extent to which Subject #1 has learned about Subject #2 involves the same general procedures as those involved in the analysis of the extent to which #1 has learned from #2. There is a difference, however, in that the test of the extent to which #1 has learned about #2 requires #1 to *predict* the judgments of #2. Once those predictions are made, the investigator may study the details of #1's inaccuracies, should they occur. That is, the investigator may ascertain whether #1 has failed to predict #2's judgments because *(a)* #1 does not *know* the manner in which #2 weights the various cues, which function forms #2 applies to them, or how #2 organizes the information; or *(b)* because #1 fails to apply his knowledge of #2 with *consistency;* or *(c)* because #2 is so *inconsistent* in his judgments that accurate prediction of his judgments would be impossible, or at least very limited for anyone. (The reader may wish to refer to (1) and the discussion following if the reasons for this analysis are not obvious.) And, as in the case of learning from the other, the question of the effect of psychoactive drugs on these aspects of learning about another person needs investigation. Such investigations are carried out in Chapters 10, 11, 12, and 13.

Although no special circumstances are required for the study of learning *from* another over and beyond the method and procedure used in studying interpersonal conflict, some additional measures are required for the study of the extent to which one person learns *about* another; these are described immediately below.

*Method and Procedure (IPL about Another).* Following the conflict phase of the research paradigm, subjects are asked to participate in a second series of trials. In this series they are asked to look at the data on a cue card, to make a judgment of the value of the criterion, and in addition to predict what judgment the other person will make in response to the same data. This is not an unreasonable request, inasmuch as the two persons have been comparing judgments with regard to these same cues for at least 20 trials, and have been discussing their judgments for roughly an hour or more.

This simple procedure produces considerable information bearing directly on the question of how much each person has learned about the other. A comparison of #1's judgment predictions for #2 with the judgments #2 made in fact provides a measure of *predictive accuracy.* In addition, it is possible to compare the predictions #1 made for #2 with #1's own judgments about the cue cards. This comparison provides a measure of *assumed similarity,* for if #1 predicts that #2 would make the same judgment that #1 made, then #1 implicitly assumes that #2 is highly similar to #1. Also, comparing #1's judgments with #2's judgments provides a measure of *actual similarity* (Brehmer, 1973; Earle, 1973; Hammond, Wilkins, & Todd, 1966).

It is possible, of course, to study the effects of various psychoactive drugs on all three measures described above. By doing so one might ascertain that a given drug increased or decreased the ability to learn about another person's judgmental system (predictive accuracy); further information could be provided by ascertaining that the increase or decrease in accuracy was obtained through a change in sensitivity to, or assumed similarity with, the difference between one's own judgmental system and that of the other's. And, of course, the extent to which each person was required to develop predictive accuracy by detecting differences in judgmental systems is indicated by the measure of actual similarity.

An alternative to the procedure described above in which the IPL phase is added to the conflict phase, is a procedure Gillis found convenient and useful in his study of schizophrenics. Because he was primarily interested in his patients' ability to learn about the other, he introduced the IPL phase directly—without a conflict phase. He simply brought persons with different judgmental systems together (by means of "policy capturing") and asked them to write down their task judgments independently and then to discuss them—without asking them to resolve the differences between their judgments. According to Gillis, this procedure worked particularly well with highly disturbed patients because it eliminated the necessity for coming to terms with the other person (see Chapter 10).

In an effort to reduce the time spent in the research situation, and because of the unstable nature of the chronic schizophrenic patients under study, Gillis also used the policy capturing procedure in the studies reported in Chapter 13.

## SUMMARY

The purpose of the present chapter is to make explicit the general theoretical and methodological context in which the empirical studies described in Part II are embedded, *but only with respect to their psychological aspects*. Nothing is said in this chapter about the relation between the psychological concepts within social judgment theory and the specific biochemical or pharmacological properties of the psychoactive drugs employed. No explicit link is made between such concepts as performance, knowledge, and control, and for example, the molecular structure of the various compounds used in the various studies, although such links should, and possibly will, be made eventually.

The principal aim of the chapter is to establish a broad theoretical framework for the systematic study of the effects of psychoactive drugs on one of man's critical functions, human judgment. A second, but no less important, aim is to illustrate what can be learned from the systematic application of social judgment theory over a series of studies. Once it has been determined that a given theory is useful—that is, that it serves its function well as a guide to organized description, quantification, and perhaps even explanation—then it may serve to direct research to more specific hypotheses concerning the biochemistry of human judgment, particularly with respect to its function in interpersonal conflict and interpersonal learning.

Social judgment theory calls attention to the importance of human judgment in social life and emphasizes the consequences of the failure to employ good judgment. A broad formulation of the process of judgment is presented, which is then interpreted quantitatively. The quantitative formulation is applied to the judgment process in three cases: learning to improve one's judgment; interpersonal conflict; and interpersonal learning. The relation between judgment in the research situations employed here and the ordinary encounters of social life is direct and obvious. Improvements are needed, however, and it is to be hoped that future investigators will find the exploratory steps taken here to be of some value.

The results of these investigations indicate that the theory did serve a useful function in organizing the description of the judgment process, in enabling the investigators to measure changes in this process as various psychoactive drugs affected it, and, occasionally, in providing explanations of what occurred. Future work may well find it appropriate to make use of the theory, both in extending our knowledge about the biochemistry of cognition, and in evaluating the effects of various psychoactive drugs prior to the attempt to apply them therapeutically.

## REFERENCES

Bandura, A. Psychotherapy based upon modeling principles. In A. E. Bergin and S. L. Garfield (Eds.), *Handbook of psychotherapy and behavior change: An empirical analysis.* New York: Wiley, 1971.

Brehmer, B. Cognitive dependence on additive and configural cue-criterion relations. *American Journal of Psychology,* 1969, **82,** 490–503.

Brehmer, B. Effects of cue validity on interpersonal learning of inference tasks with linear and nonlinear cues. *American Journal of Psychology,* 1973, **86,** 29–48.

Brehmer, B. and Hammond, K. R. Cognitive sources of interpersonal conflict. Analysis of interactions between linear and nonlinear cognitive systems. *Organizational Behavior and Human Performance,* 1973, **10,** 290–313.

Brunswik, E. *Perception and the representative design of psychological experiments.* Berkeley, California: University of California Press, 1956.

Brunswik, E. Reasoning as a universal behavior model and a functional differentiation between "perception" and "thinking." In K. R. Hammond (Ed.), *The psychology of Egon Brunswik.* New York: Holt, Rinehart & Winston, 1966.

Cvetkovich, G. Small group dynamics in extended judgment situations. In L. Rappoport and D. Summers (Eds.), *Human judgment and social interaction.* New York: Holt, Rinehart & Winston, 1973.

Deane, D. H., Hammond, K. R., and Summers, D. A. Acquisition and application of knowledge in complex inference tasks. *Journal of Experimental Psychology,* 1972, **92,** 20–26.

Earle, T. C. Interpersonal learning. In L. Rappoport and D. Summers (Eds.), *Human judgment and social interaction.* New York: Holt, Rinehart & Winston, 1973.

Goldberg, L. R. Man versus model of man: A rationale, plus some evidence for a method of improving on clinical inferences. *Psychological Bulletin,* 1970, **73,** 422–432.

Hammond, K. R. New directions in research on conflict resolution. *Journal of Social Issues,* 1965, **21,** 44–66.

Hammond, K. R. Probabilistic functionalism: Egon Brunswik's integration of the history, theory, and method of psychology. In K. R. Hammond (Ed.), *The psychology of Egon Brunswik.* New York: Holt, Rinehart & Winston, 1966.

Hammond, K. R. Computer graphics as an aid to learning. *Science,* 1971, **172,** 903–908.

Hammond, K. R. Inductive knowing. In J. R. Royce and W. N. Rozeboom (Eds.), *The psychology of knowing.* London: Gordon & Breach, 1972.

Hammond, K. R. and Boyle, P. J. R. Quasi-rationality, quarrels and new conceptions of feedback. *Bulletin of the British Psychological Society,* 1971, **24,** 103–113.

Hammond, K. R. and Brehmer, B. Quasi-rationality and distrust: Implications for international conflict. In L. Rappoport and D. Summers (Eds.), *Human judgment and social interaction*. New York: Holt, Rinehart & Winston, 1973.

Hammond, K. R., Stewart, T. R., Brehmer, B., and Steinmann, D. O. Social Judgment Theory. In M. F. Kaplan and S. Schwartz (Eds.), *Human judgment and decision processes: Formal and mathematical approaches*. New York: Academic Press, 1975.

Hammond, K. R., and Summers, D. A. Cognitive dependence on linear and nonlinear cues. *Psychological Review*, 1965, **72**, 215–224.

Hammond, K. R. and Summers, D. A. Cognitive control. *Psychological Review*, 1972, **79**, 58–67.

Hammond, K. R., Wilkins, M., and Todd, F. J. A research paradigm for the study of interpersonal learning. *Psychological Bulletin*, 1966, **65**, 221–232.

Hursch, C., Hammond, K. R., and Hursch, J. Some methodological considerations in multiple-cue probability studies. *Psychological Review*, 1964, **71**, 42–60.

Kessel, C. Effects of group pressure and commitment on conflict, adaptability, and cognitive change. In L. Rappoport and D. Summers (Eds.), *Human judgment and social interaction*. New York: Holt, Rinehart & Winston, 1973.

Moscovici, S., Lage, E., and Naffrechoux, M. Conflict in three-person groups: The relationship between social influence and cognitive style. In L. Rappoport and D. Summers (Eds.), *Human judgment and social interaction*. New York: Holt, Rinehart & Winston, 1973.

Rappoport, L. Cognitive conflict as a function of socially-induced cognitive differences. *Journal of Conflict Resolution*, 1969, **13**, 143–148.

Slovic, P. and Lichtenstein, S. Comparison of Bayesian and regression approaches to the study of information processing in judgment. In L. Rappoport and D. Summers (Eds.), *Human judgment and social interaction*. New York: Holt, Rinehart & Winston, 1973.

Stewart, T. R. Components of correlations and extensions of the lens model equation. Unpublished manuscript, University of Colorado, Institute of Behavioral Science, Program of Research on Human Judgment and Social Interaction, Report No. 146, 1973.

Summers, D. A. and Hammond, K. R. Inference behavior in multiple-cue tasks involving both linear and nonlinear relations. *Journal of Experimental Psychology*, 1966, **71**, 751–757.

Tucker, L. R. A suggested alternative formulation in the developments by Hursch, Hammond, and Hursch, and by Hammond, Hursch and Todd. *Psychological Review*, 1964, **71**, 528–530.

Webster's 2nd International Dictionary (unabridged).

## Articles on Interpersonal Conflict

Adelman, L., Stewart, T. R., and Hammond, K. R. A case history of the application of social judgment theory to policy formulation, *Policy Sciences*, 1975, **6**, 137–159.

Balke, W. M., Hammond, K. R., and Meyer, G. D. An alternative approach to labor-management negotiations. *Administrative Science Quarterly*, 1973, **18**, 311–327.

Bonaiuto, G. B. The feedback problem: Cognitive change in conditions of exact and ambiguous outcome information. In L. Rappoport and D. Summers (Eds.), *Human judgment and social interaction*. New York: Holt, Rinehart & Winston, 1973.

Brehmer, B. The roles of policy differences and inconsistency in policy conflict. *Umea Psychological Reports* No. 18, 1969, and University of Colorado, Institute of Behavioral Science, Program of Research on Human Judgment and Social Interaction Report No. 118, 1969.

Brehmer, B. Kommunikation och konflikt. In M. Bjorkman and I. Lunaberg (Eds.), *Fordjupningstexter Till Psykologi For Gymnasiet*. Stockholm, Almqvist and Wiksell, 1970. *(a)*

Brehmer, B. Sequence effects in policy conflict. *Umea Psychological Reports* No. 17, 1969, and University of Colorado, Institute of Behavioral Science, Program of Research on Human Judgment and Social Interaction Report No. 133, 1970. *(b)*

Brehmer, B. The structure of policy conflict. *Umea Psychological Reports* No. 29, 1970. *(c)*

Brehmer, B. Effects of communication and feedback on cognitive conflict. *Scandinavian Journal of Psychology*, 1971, **12**, 205–216.

Brehmer, B. Policy conflict as a function of policy similarity and policy complexity. *Scandinavian Journal of Psychology*, 1972, **13**, 208–221.

Brehmer, B. Policy conflict and policy change as a function of task characteristics: II. The effect of task predictability. *Scandinavian Journal of Psychology*, 1973, **14**, 220–227. *(a)*

Brehmer, B. Policy conflict, policy consistency, and interpersonal understanding. *Umea Psychological Reports* No. 71, 1973. *(b)*

Brehmer, B. Policy conflict and policy change as a function of task characteristics: III. The effects of the distribution of the validities of the cues in the conflict task. *Scandinavian Journal of Psychology*, 1974, **15**, 135–138.

Brehmer, B., Azuma, H., Hammond, K. R., Kostron, L., and Varonos, D. D. A cross-cultural comparison of cognitive conflict. *Journal of Cross-Cultural Psychology*, 1970, **1**, 5–20.

Brehmer, B., and Garpebring, S. Social pressure and policy change in the "Lens Model" interpersonal conflict paradigm. *Scandinavian Journal of Psychology*, 1974, **15**, 191–196.

Brehmer, B. and Hammond, K. R. Cognitive sources of interpersonal conflict. Analysis of interactions between linear and nonlinear cognitive systems. *Organizational Behavior and Human Performance*, 1973, **10**, 290–313.

Brehmer, B. and Kostron, L. Policy conflict and policy change as a function of task characteristics: I. The effects of cue validity and function form. *Scandinavian Journal of Psychology*, 1973, **14**, 44–55.

Earle, T. Task learning, interpersonal learning, and cognitive complexity. *Oregon Research Institute Research Bulletin*, 1970, **10**, 2.

Earle, T. Interpersonal learning. In L. Rappoport and D. Summers (Eds.), *Human judgment and social interaction*. New York: Holt, Rinehart & Winston, 1973.

Flack, J. E. and Summers, D. A. Computer aided conflict resolution in water resource planning: An illustration. *Water Resources Research*, 1971, **7**, 1410–1414.

Hammond, K. R. New directions in research on conflict resolution. *Journal of Social Issues*, 1965, **21**, 44–66.

Hammond, K. R. The cognitive conflict paradigm. In L. Rappoport and D. Summers (Eds.), *Human judgment and social interaction*. New York: Holt, Rinehart & Winston, 1973. *(a)*

Hammond, K. R. White collar conflict. *Social Education*, 1973, **37**, 627–629. *(b)*

Hammond, K. R. and Boyle, P. J. R. Quasi-rationality, quarrels and new conceptions of feedback. *Bulletin of the British Psychological Society*, 1971, **24**, 103–113.

Hammond, K. R. and Brehmer, B. Quasi-rationality and distrust: Implications for international conflict. In L. Rappoport and D. Summers (Eds.), *Human judgment and social interaction*. New York: Holt, Rinehart & Winston, 1973.

Hammond, K. R., Todd, F. J., Wilkins, M., and Mitchell, T. O. Cognitive conflict between persons: Application of the "lens model" paradigm. *Journal of Experimental Social Psychology*, 1966, **2**, 343–360.

Helenius, M. Socially induced cognitive conflict: A study of disagreement over childrearing policies. In L. Rappoport and D. Summers (Eds.), *Human judgment and social interaction*. New York: Holt, Rinehart & Winston, 1973.

Kuhlman, C., Miller, M. J., and Gungor, E. Interpersonal conflict reduction: The effects of language and meaning. In L. Rappoport and D. Summers (Eds.), *Human judgment and social interaction*. New York: Holt, Rinehart & Winston, 1973.

Miller, M. J., Brehmer, B., and Hammond, K. R. Communication and conflict reduction: A cross-cultural study. *International Journal of Psychology*, 1970, **5**, 75–87.

Mumpower, J. L. and Hammond, K. R. Entangled task-dimensions: An impediment to interpersonal learning. *Organizational Behavior and Human Performance*, 1974, **11**, 377–389.

Rappoport, L. Cognitive conflict as a function of socially induced cognitive differences. *Journal of Conflict Resolution*, 1969, **13**, 143–148.

Summers, D. A. Conflict, compromise, and belief change in a decision-making task. *Journal of Conflict Resolution*, 1968, **2**, 215–221.

Todd, F. J., Hammond, K. R., and Wilkins, M. Differential effects of ambiguous and exact feedback on two-person conflict and compromise. *Journal of Conflict Resolution*, 1966, **10**, 88–97.

# PART TWO

# Empirical Studies

Pharmacological aids in the form of psychoactive drugs are widely used in the control of social behavior of psychotic persons, and widely accepted by psychiatrists, other physicians, and lay persons as aids to the reduction of depression, fatigue, or anxiety, or as facilitators of social interaction, despite the fact that little is known about the specific details of the functional relations between the biochemistry of such drugs and behavior. Despite the large areas of ignorance, there is definite reason to believe that changes in the biochemistry of the nervous system do produce changes in cognitive activity (see Chapters 1 and 2). The studies in Part II address the question of whether the biochemical changes produced in the nervous system by certain well-known psychoactive drugs lead to changes in those critical cognitive functions involved in the exercise of social judgment. These studies are concerned with the effects of such drugs on the ability to learn to improve one's judgment, as well as their effects on cognitive abilities in situations where quarrels arise from differing judgments and in situations requiring interpersonal learning. These are the situations in which failures of judgment are quickly detected, and from which conclusions are drawn about the extent to which a person is a danger to himself and others.

CHAPTER 4

# Effects of Chlorpromazine and Thiothixene on Acute Schizophrenic Patients

JOHN S. GILLIS

It has been recognized for several years that although certain antipsychotic drugs yield important benefits in symptom alleviation, they seem to impair rather than facilitate learning. The data are most abundant and most dramatic with regard to chlorpromazine. Hartlage, after reviewing numerous studies of the drug's effect on learning in animals and humans, could conclude that "... since chlorpromazine is consensually considered the drug of choice for treatment of schizophrenic disorders . . . such treatment must be willing to sacrifice some degree of learning on the part of the patient [1965, p. 241]." The conclusion is an important one; regardless of how one conceives of psychological therapies, they obviously involve the patient's learning something—whether this be altered behaviors, more adaptive attitudes, or new insights into himself and his situation. If the price paid for symptom control is a seriously diminished capacity for learning, it may be a high price indeed.

Initial studies of the effects of chlorpromazine on the ability to learn to make judgments have been generally congruent with the larger body of learning data. Thus Davis, Evans, and Gillis (1969) found that chlorpromazine impaired the judgmental learning of normal college students. Gillis and Davis (1973), using a hospitalized chronic schizophrenic sample, found a similar deleterious effect of chlorpromazine when compared to methamphetamine.

These studies have been exploratory, of course, and were limited both by the subject samples involved and the failure to include antipsychotic agents other than chlorpromazine. They were also based on single administrations of drugs rather than administrations over a prolonged period of time. The present investigation sought to broaden the study of the effects of antipsychotic drugs on judgmental learning in regard to both matters. Therefore, acute adolescent schizophrenics were employed, and a second antipsychotic agent, not in the phenothiazine group, was included.

The drugs selected were chlorpromazine (Thorazine) and thiothixene (Navane). The former was chosen as a representative of the phenothiazines because of (1) its widespread use with schizophrenics, (2) the substantial body of evidence already available regarding its clinical efficacy (Klein & Davis, 1969), (3) its negative implications for learning (Hartlage, 1965), and (4) effects on performance previously found with materials similar to those used in this study (Davis, Evans, & Gillis, 1969; Gillis & Davis, 1973). Thiothixene, a thioxanthene derivative, was selected because it is a major antipsychotic agent, not in the phenothiazine group, that has been demonstrated to be effective in the reduction of schizophrenic symptoms and appears to be especially useful for symptoms involving social withdrawal.

The investigation described was part of a larger study of the effects of antipsychotic drugs on human judgment.


## METHOD

Adolescent acute schizophrenics received one of two antipsychotic drugs or a placebo over a period of two weeks, after which time they completed a series of tasks that involved (1) learning to improve judgments with regard to objective tasks, (2) attempting to resolve cognitive differences with another person, and (3) learning about another individual. Performance of the drug and placebo groups was compared on a variety of indices described below. These included measures of achievement and its components (knowledge and control) in each of the three judgmental situations, as well as indices specific to task learning, conflict resolution, and interpersonal learning.

This chapter presents the results regarding objective task learning, and describes the characteristics of the tasks and procedures utilized. Chapter 7 describes the results—obtained with the same drugs, patients, and procedures—with regard to conflict reduction. Chapter 10 summarizes the data obtained on interpersonal learning. In both of these chapters the reader is referred to the present chapter for details concerning method and procedure. Finally, although a summary of results is given in each of the three chapters, a full discussion of the findings is withheld until all results have been considered (Chapter 13).

## PROCEDURE

### Drugs

Subjects were randomly assigned to one of the three treatment groups. Group A received 300 mg of chlorpromazine (75 mg, q.i.d.) daily; Group B, 20 mg thiothixene (5 mg, q.i.d.) daily; and Group C, a lactose placebo. Medications and placebo were packaged identically and were administered by ward nursing personnel as a part of their standard medication routines.

All subjects were on the experimental regimens for 14 days; no "wash-out" period was used. Although the maximally desirable conditions for this investigation would include (1) a longer duration of treatment before testing and (2) a "wash-out" period, the 14-day treatment period appeared to be sufficient to test the social and cognitive effects of interest, without unduly disturbing a ward for acutely disturbed patients.

### Subjects

The subjects were 19 acute schizophrenic patients resident in a ward for severely disturbed adolescents at Mendocino State Hospital, California. This group included both paranoid ($n = 10$) and nonparanoid ($n = 9$) patients, the diagnostic distinction being made by using Venables' scale for rating paranoid schizophrenia (Venables & O'Connor, 1959). Ages ranged from 14 to 19, the mean age being 16.8 years. IQ, measured by the Otis Alpha Test, ranged from 80 to 121, with 12 of the 19 subjects falling in the range 85–99. Educational level ranged from grade 6 through 12 with 14 of the subjects having completed 9–11 years of school. Gillis and Davis (1973) had found that neither IQ nor educational level related significantly to performance on tasks similar to those used in this investigation. However, the three treatment groups were matched for age, IQ, and educational attainment.

Subjects were not included in the study if there were any indications of organic brain damage or any history of excessive drug use. Patients about whom there was disagreement as to diagnosis were also excluded.

Once selected for the study, subjects were randomly assigned to one of the three experimental groups—chlorpromazine (CPZ), thiothixene, or placebo—and received the appropriate medication according to the schedule described. After 12 days on the psychoactive drugs or placebo, subjects were administered one of two forms of a judgmental learning task, the details of which are described below. After 14 days on the drug treatment regimen, subjects participated in the conflict and interpersonal learning (IPL) tasks (also described in detail below).

Since the conflict-IPL tasks required subjects to work in pairs, it was necessary to select a partner for each member of the experimental groups. The analysis of the results would have been facilitated if all subjects could have worked with partners receiving the same treatment; that is, if all CPZ subjects could have worked with other members of the CPZ treatment group. Such an arrangement of partners was not possible, however, because of practical considerations. Chief among these was the brief hospital stay of many patients; that is, if patient X did not start on his treatment until a potential partner was available, he might well be discharged before he could be used in the study at all. This being the case, any patient eligible (according to the diagnostic and intelligence criteria mentioned) was immediately assigned to a treatment. When each was due to work on the conflict-IPL tasks (after 14 days on treatment), his partner was selected from available patients on the "acutely disturbed adolescent" program. In almost all cases (16 of 19), this partner was also a schizophrenic, but in only 3 of the 19 pairs was he a member of the same drug treatment group.

In short, in the tasks requiring patient interaction, partners for the subjects in any of the three drug treatment groups might be patients from *(a)* the same treatment group, *(b)* from another of the treatment groups, or *(c)* not in the study at all, although resident in the same ward. When discussing the performance of, let us say, chlorpromazine subjects on the interactive tasks, we will, therefore, be considering how these patients performed with a sample of partners heterogeneous as far as the drug treatment is concerned. Despite the primarily practical grounds requiring such heterogeneity, this manner of selecting partners might also be said to constitute a more representative sample of the kinds of individuals with whom these subjects would interact during their hospitalization. Adequate representation of the ecology has always been a major requirement of research in the Brunswikian framework (Brunswik, 1955, 1956; Hammond, 1965), and its lack of studies of pathological populations is a serious drawback to the meaningfulness of such studies. The presence of a varied group of partners in the assessment of drug effects on social interaction and interpersonal learning, therefore, is a strength rather than a weakness in the current investigation.

In summary, the design of the study called for random assignment to one of three treatment conditions—thiothixene, chlorpromazine, or placebo. Subjects remained on the experimental treatment for 14 days. After 12 days they completed a judgmental learning task. After 14 days they worked with partners, selected from a variety of acutely disturbed adolescent patients, in a situation that allowed the investigators to assess capacity of these patients to resolve conflicts and to learn from and about another person.

## Description of Tasks

The tasks were similar to those used by Gillis in several studies of complex learning with schizophrenics (Gillis, 1969, 1971; Gillis & Davis, 1973). The judgmental learning tasks provide subjects with a variety of cues, each having an uncertain relationship with the criterion. They must learn to utilize the cues effectively to infer the correct value of the criterion variable. Two forms of these tasks were used, varying along a continuum of what has been referred to as "wide" and "narrow" focusing (Gillis & Davis, 1973). Tasks that demand the use of only a single cue, or a limited number of cues, are referred to as "narrow-focus" tasks; those requiring the integration of several cues are termed "wide-focus." This dimension had been found useful in differentiating among subtypes (paranoid and nonparanoid) of schizophrenics as well as among selected psychoactive chemicals (Gillis & Davis, 1973; Davis, Evans, & Gillis, 1969).

In each judgmental learning task used in this study there were three cues; each was related in a linear, probabilistic way to the criterion. In the narrow-focus task *(A)*, only one cue had any significant predictive validity, the other two cues having near zero correlations with the criterion. In the wide-focus task *(B)*, each had a significant and roughly equal predictive validity. In order to perform successfully on task *A*, subjects needed only to learn to take into account a single item of information when making their responses. Their performance, in fact, would be impaired to the extent that they utilized the other cues. To perform successfully in the wide-focus task *(B)*, however, subjects had to take into account all available information contained in the three cues. It was not possible in either task for a subject to be perfectly correct on every trial; that is, the multiple correlation $R^2$ controlling both tasks was approximately .85. The statistical properties of the tasks are summarized in Figure 4.1.

### Details of the Judgmental Learning Tasks

The task materials consisted of 10-point scales (cues) printed on cards, each of which indicated the value of the cue by the height of a vertical black bar. These cues were related to the criterion according to one of the two correlational structures described above.

Subjects were informed that the correct answer was a number on the back of the card that ranged from 1 to 20 and could be predicted with considerable, although

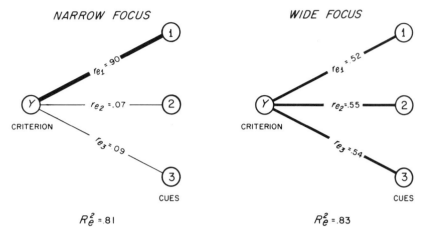

**Figure 4.1.**    Statistical structures of the judgmental learning tasks.

not perfect, accuracy from the cues on the front of the card. It was also explained that the cue values varied, and that these values were represented by the height of the bar. After being given three illustrative practice trials, all subjects were shown the first cue card, and then asked to record their predictions of the correct answer on their response sheets. Following this prediction they were immediately informed of the right answer. This immediate outcome feedback was the only kind of feedback given throughout the 80 trial learning tasks. (See Chapter 14 for a description of the performance of schizophrenic patients when cognitive feedback, described in Chapter 3, is provided.)

## RESULTS AND DISCUSSION

### Measures of Performance

*Achievement*

Performance on the judgmental learning tasks was assessed by correlating subject's responses over trials with the correct answers. These achievement correlation coefficients $r_a$ were calculated for eight blocks of 10 trials each and then transformed into Fisher's z-scores for subsequent statistical analysis. The resulting scores for the narrow- and wide-focus tasks and for all three treatment groups (Figures 4.2 and 4.3) indicate that achievement (that is, learning) was greatest for the placebo group in both tasks (the main effect for drug groups over both tasks yielded an $F$ ratio of 12.86; $df = 2,11$; $p < .01$). Although the thiothixene group was more effective than the chlorpromazine group in the

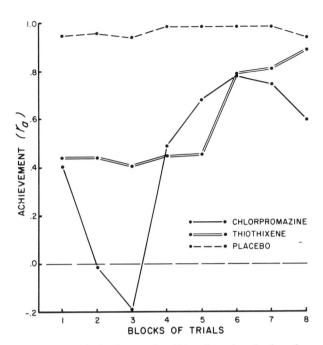

**Figure 4.2.** Achievement $r_a$ in the "narrow-focus" learning task under three drug conditions.

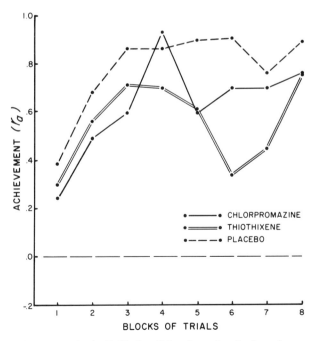

**Figure 4.3** Achievement $r_a$ in the "wide-focus" learning task under three drug conditions.

narrow-focus task, the achievement level acquired by the two drug groups was roughly the same, and both were slightly inferior to placebo subjects on the wide-focus task.

## Knowledge

Hammond (Chapter 3) has already discussed the value of analyzing performance in learning tasks in terms of knowledge $G$ and control $R$. The knowledge measure $G$ represents the extent to which a subject's cognitive system is isomorphic with the task system, independent of the uncertainty in both systems. The value of $G$ was determined for each of the treatment groups and for both task situations. Results (Figures 4.4 and 4.5) parallel those for achievement. There are significant and main effects for blocks of trials ($F = 2.18$; $df = 7, 77$; $p < .05$) and drug groups ($F = 11.81$; $df = 2, 11$; $p < .01$). Again, placebo subjects perform most effectively and chlorpromazine subjects least effectively, and again these differences are most pronounced in the narrow-focus task.

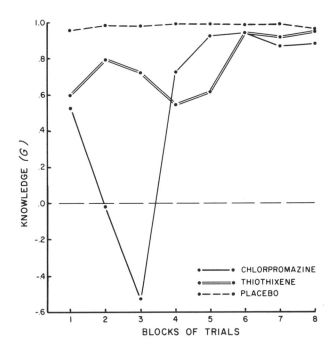

**Figure 4.4.** Knowledge $G$ in the "narrow-focus" learning task under three drug conditions.

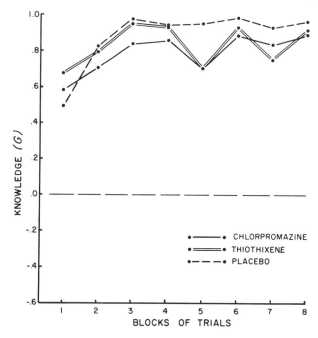

**Figure 4.5.** Knowledge $G$ in the "wide-focus" learning task under three drug conditions.

## Consistency

The measure of consistency for the judgmental learning tasks and also for the interaction tasks is $R^2$; that is, the squared multiple correlation between the $n$ sources of information (the three cues) with which a subject is confronted and the judgments he makes. This index is plotted for the narrow-focus task in Figure 4.6 and for the wide-focus task in Figure 4.7. The order of consistency among the treatment groups was the same as the order of achievement—placebo subjects were the most consistent and CPZ subjects were least consistent, the thiothixene group falling between the two. There were essentially no differences among the groups on the wide-focus task, although the subjects in the placebo group were again somewhat more consistent than those in either of the drug groups.

The clearest findings were in the narrow-focus task (Figure 4.2) where the cue-criterion correlations were .9, .1, .1, and which prior studies (Gillis, 1969; Gillis & Davis, 1973) have indicated is less difficult for schizophrenic subjects. Perhaps the most impressive aspect of the results on this task is that the achievement level of the placebo group of patients did not differ greatly from that of the college students confronted with a very similar task in an earlier study (Gillis,

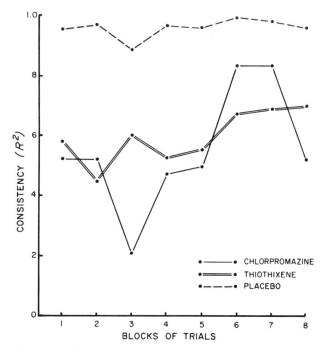

**Figure 4.6.** Consistency $R^2$ in the "narrow-focus" learning task under three drug conditions.

1969). These schizophrenic patients, therefore, performed as well as bright normals on tasks where the use of only a limited amount of information is required.

Such task structures may, in fact, be less difficult for nonparanoid schizophrenics than for normals because the task structure is compatible with the cognitive styles of such patients. Thus, the results suggest support for the general argument by Gillis and Davis (1973) that schizophrenics can be termed "cognitively impaired" only in regard to specific structures.

Although schizophrenics receiving placebos can deal effectively with "narrow-focus" tasks, their ability to do so is diminished when tranquilizing drugs are given. One possible explanation for this is that chlorpromazine and thiothixene enhance the alertness of recipients, thus causing them to take account of more cues. This kind of cognitive-perceptual style, or approach to multiple-cue tasks, would be maladaptive in the narrow-focus circumstance, although perhaps more useful in coping with tasks ordinarily encountered. In order to investigate this possibility, the cue-utilization patterns of the three treatment groups were evaluated for the narrow-focus task. If, in fact, disruption of narrow-focus performance were due to attending to more than the one valid cue, the responses of subjects treated with drugs should correlate highly with the invalid cues.

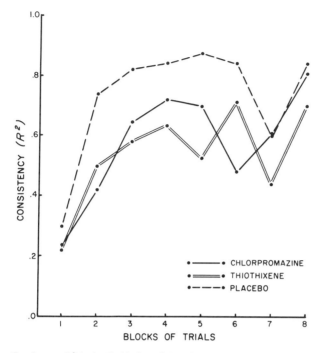

**Figure 4.7.**    Consistency $R^2$ in the "wide-focus" learning task under three drug conditions.

Such was not the case, however; the drug-treated groups did not use invalid cues more than the placebo subjects did. Rather than focusing on more than one cue, the subjects receiving drugs were simply less effective in their use of the single important cue. "Less effective" means, in large part, less consistent. As Figure 4.6 indicates, the order of levels of consistency $R^2$ among the treatment groups paralleled their achievement $r_a$. The impaired performance of the drug groups, particularly the chlorpromazine subjects, seems, therefore, to have been the result of an inconsistent way of dealing with the task rather than increased attention and responsiveness to a number of cues.

The difficulty of the wide-focus task (cue-criterion correlations of .5, .5, .5) noted in previous learning studies (Gillis, 1969; Gillis & Davis, 1973) is perhaps responsible for obscuring differences among the treatment groups. Placebo subjects do, however, again demonstrate somewhat higher achievement and greater consistency than do either of the drug groups.

The results supplement previous findings (Gillis & Davis, 1973; Hartlage, 1965) that chlorpromazine impairs cognitive functioning without regard to the complexity of the learning situations. When not receiving either of the drugs studied here, however, even these acutely disturbed schizophrenics performed at a level approximating that of normals with regard to learning and improved judgment. The findings thus support Hartlage's contention that, while chlorpromazine is definitely associated with symptom reduction, a significant decrease in a patient's ability to learn may have to be accepted as a consequence of that treatment. An equally important possibility is that the negative effect on learning may be characteristic of antipsychotic drugs other than chlorpromazine. Information bearing on this very critical point will come from extensions of the kind of study reported here.

## REFERENCES

Brunswik, E. Representative design and probabilistic theory in a functional psychology. *Psychological Review*, 1955, **62,** 193–217.

Brunswik, E. *Perception and the representative design of experiments*. Berkeley: University of California Press, 1956.

Davis, K. E., Evans, W. O., and Gillis, J. S. The effects of amphetamine and chlorpromazine on cognitive skills and feelings in normal adult males. In W. O. Evans and N. Kline (Eds.), *The psychopharmacology of the normal human*. Springfield, Ill.: Charles C. Thomas, 1969.

Gillis, J. S. Schizophrenic thinking is a probabilistic situation. *Psychological Record*, 1969, **19,** 211–224.

Gillis, J. S. Ecological relevance and the study of diversed thinking. In J. Hellmuth (Ed.), *Cognitive studies*, Vol. 2: *Deficits in cognition*. New York: Brunner-Mazel, 1971.

Gillis, J. S. and Davis, K. E. The effects of psychoactive drugs on complex thinking in paranoid and nonparanoid schizophrenics: An application of the multiple-cue model to the study of disordered thinking. In L. Rappoport and D. Summers (Eds.), *Human judgment and social interaction*. New York: Holt, Rinehart & Winston, 1973.

Hammond, K. R. New directions in research on conflict resolution. *Journal of Social Issues*, 1965, **21,** 44–66.

Hartlage, L. C. Effects of chlorpromazine on learning. *Psychological Bulletin*, 1965, **64,** 235–245.

Klein, D. F. and Davis, J. M. *Diagnosis and drug treatment of psychiatric disorders*. Baltimore: Williams and Wilkins, 1969.

Venables, P. H. and O'Connor, N. A. A short scale for rating paranoid schizophrenia. *The Journal of Mental Science*, 1959, **105,** 815–818.

CHAPTER 5

# Effects of Methylphenidate on Mildly Depressed Hospitalized Adults

ELLEN R. GRITZ

This experiment measured the effect of a psychoactive drug on the ability of mildly depressed patients to learn to improve their judgment. The effects of psychoactive agents upon cognitive functions have been analyzed both clinically and experimentally (see Chapters 1 and 2). The more global clinical assessments usually rely upon interviews, rating scales, and subjective impressions of improvement or deterioration. Experimental evaluations of changes in intellectual processes, or subsidiary functions of attention and perception, generally utilize tests developed in the psychological laboratory, for example, verbal learning, signal detection tasks, or tests with motor involvement. The experimental evaluation of the effect of such drugs upon intellectual functioning with regard to the exercise of judgment is undertaken in this volume.

Centrally acting sympathomimetic amines have been frequently considered as facilitators of intellectual functioning. In a review of the effects of amphetamine and caffeine, however, Weiss and Laties (1962) concluded that these drugs probably enhanced physical performance and aggravated fatigue, but did not enhance intellectual performance. Herrington (1967) found that amphetamine reduced the number of errors made on a choice serial reaction task; however, decline in performance over time (fatigue effect) did not differentiate drug and placebo groups. Likewise, Talland and Quarton (1966) found that methamphetamine, compared to saline, increased the number of correct responses in signal detection, which they attributed to an improvement in sustained attention and not to reduced fatigue. Whether methamphetamine actually produces any direct effects upon attention is still open to question. Callaway (1959) maintains that the Stroop test (color reading and color naming requiring an unusual perceptual set) measures the narrowing, or focus of attention. He obtained facilitation of

121

performance with methamphetamine, among other drugs. Quarton and Talland (1962) failed to replicate Callaway's findings and also obtained no effect of methamphetamine upon the running digit span, a measure of attention and short-term storage of stimuli (Talland and Quarton, 1965). It appears, therefore, that no firm claims can be made for the effects of amphetamine on any type of intellectual process so far examined.

Empirical findings regarding mood effects are somewhat clearer. Methamphetamine and methylphenidate produce euphoric feelings of contentment and proficiency in adults when low and moderate doses are used; nervousness appears only at high doses (Martin, Sloan, Sapira, & Jasinski, 1971). Methylphenidate, itself, is described pharmacologically as an analeptic, a piperidine derivative, which probably acts by enhancing synaptic excitation. ''The drug is a mild CNS (central nervous system) stimulant, more effective than caffeine but less effective than amphetamine in increasing motor and mental activities. Respiration and blood pressure are little affected by doses of methylphenidate that produce CNS stimulation [Esplin and Zablocka-Esplin, 1970, p. 354].''

The stimulants, particularly methylphenidate, have been used therapeutically for hyperkinetic children with gross behavioral disturbances and severe learning disorders. The ''paradoxical'' calming effect on behavior and improvement in learning ability produced by stimulants in these children (Weiss, Minde, Douglas, Werry, & Sykes, 1971; Conners, Eisenberg, & Sharpe, 1964; Sykes, Douglas, & Morgenstern, 1972) has been attributed to increased duration of attention and lesser distractability, accompanied by more control and direction of physical activity.

If increases in attention and concentration as well as improvement in learning ability do characterize the stimulants in children, it would be reasonable to inquire whether methylphenidate could produce an improvement in the ability of adults to form judgments. The mood elevating effects of the drug on a mildly depressed patient sample might either directly facilitate judgment through central nervous system drug effects on cognitive mechanisms, or indirectly facilitate judgment by improving attention and concentration.

## METHOD

Patients with a diagnosis of mild depression were randomly assigned to either of two treatment conditions: drug (methylphenidate hydrochloride), or placebo in a double-blind design. After five days on these regimens, patients dealt with a judgment task involving both learning and interactive stages. Drug groups were compared on several indices derived from these tasks including overall achievement, knowledge of task characteristics, and cognitive control (consistency). (See Chapter 3.) Drug actions on affect were also assessed using a mood scale.

## PROCEDURE

### Subjects

Twenty-eight male patients, with a mean age of 40 (range 20–58) and a diagnosis of mild depression (some with accompanying alcoholism), were selected from new admissions to the Brentwood Veterans Administration Hospital. None were receiving major psychoactive medications; in some cases mild tranquilizers were prescribed. Subjects were assigned randomly to either of two conditions described below; there were 14 patients in each condition. Subjects were given canteen books as a reward for participation.

### Drugs

Subjects received drug or placebo on a double-blind design for 5 days; methylphenidate hydrochloride (Ritalin) 10 mg, t.i.d., or placebo t.i.d., given one-half hour before meals.

### Tasks

The tasks used were identical to those "teacher tasks" described by Gillis (Chapters 4 and 7) and are only briefly summarized here.

The subjects were required to learn to judge the effectiveness of teachers. Sets of 5 x 8 cards contained two scales (vertical bars); one bar was labeled "Intelligence" and the other was labeled "Leniency." These bars covaried with the "answer" according to the function form specified by the experimental design. Each deck consisted of 60 such cards, with varying heights of the bars. The subject's task was to evaluate "teachers" on the basis of their intelligence (linearly related to the criterion) and leniency (nonlinearly related to the criterion by an inverted U-shaped function). Subjects received outcome feedback during the learning stage; that is, for each card presented, they were told the "correct answer" after making their own judgment. (For the purposes of the studies concerning interpersonal conflict and interpersonal learning—described in Chapters 7, 8, 9, 10, 11, 12, and 13—each subject was allowed as many trials as necessary until a correlation of at least .75 with the relevant cue and no larger correlation than .25 with the irrelevant cue was reached.)

The learning task required about 1½ hours; it took place on day 4 of administration of the compounds. (The conflict and interpersonal learning sessions took place on day 5.)

## Multiple Affect Adjective Checklist (MAACL)

This instrument (Zuckerman & Lubin, 1965) is a 135-item self-report checklist from which scores for anxiety, depression, and hostility are derived, and it is generally described as a "mood scale." It was given three times: before medication was begun; on day 4 at the start of the learning session; and on day 5 at the start of the interaction session.

## RESULTS

Evaluation of learning was made in terms of the subject's performance in the first 60 trials, taken as three blocks of 20 trials. Definitions and details of calculating the several indices in this section are described in Chapter 3.

## Achievement $r_a$

A significant main effect for trial blocks demonstrated increasing dependence on the strong cue as learning progressed; subjects, that is, learned to depend on the cue correlated most highly with the criterion and to ignore the weak one. Although no significant differences in achievement occurred between drug groups or type of subject, the methylphenidate linear subjects performed consistently below the level of the placebo linear subjects and the methylphenidate nonlinear subjects performed below the other three groups over the first 40 trials (see Figure 5.1).

## Knowledge $G$

As in the measure of achievement, learning was statistically demonstrated by a significant main effect for blocks. Just as subjects came to achieve at a higher level

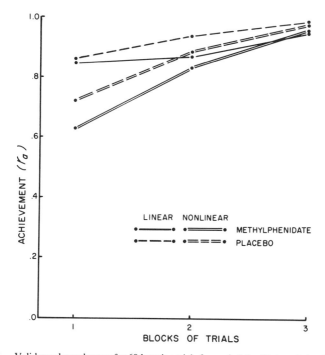

**Figure 5.1.**   Valid cue dependency $r$ for 60 learning trials for methylphenidate and placebo groups.

as trials progressed, so increasingly they were able to detect the critical characteristics of the task. Among the four subgroups, poorest performance on this measure occurred in the methylphenidate nonlinear subjects. Although the finding is nonsignificant, it is the same trend as appeared in the analysis of $r_a$ (see Figure 5.2).

## Consistency $R^2$

All subjects became significantly more consistent in making judgments over the 60 learning trials. There was a nonsignificant trend for poorer performance in methylphenidate linear trained subjects, who performed below their placebo linear counterparts (see Figure 5.3).

## Invalid Cue

In this measure, as in all other measures, subjects did improve over trial blocks. In general, subjects learning the linear cue function form reduced dependence on the

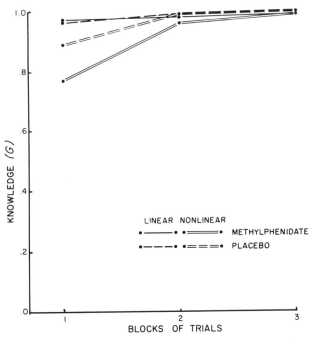

**Figure 5.2.** Knowledge $G$ for 60 learning trials for methylphenidate and placebo groups.

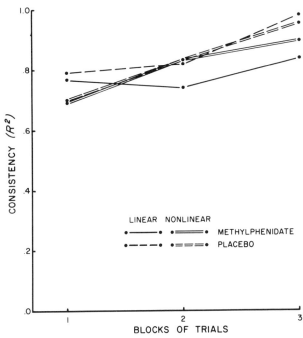

**Figure 5.3.** Consistency $R^2$ for 60 learning trials for methylphenidate and placebo groups.

invalid cue (cue-to-be-ignored) significantly more quickly than did subjects learning the nonlinear function form. Linear and nonlinear subjects did not maintain a uniform order of improvement, however; there was a significant Block by Subject interaction $(F = 3.256; df = 2, 48; p < .05)$. Although the drug group differences were not significant, the methylphenidate linear subjects did not reduce dependency on the invalid cue evenly, and the methylphenidate nonlinear subjects again performed most poorly among all subjects (see Figure 5.4).

## Learning Behavior

A clear difference between the two groups may be seen in Figure 5.5 $(F = 6.44; df = 1,24; p < .05)$, which depicts the subjects' behavior over the first 60 learning trials in terms of the subjects' decreasing dependence on the cue-to-be-ignored and increasing dependence on the valid cue. The ratio of the difference between the value of the valid cue and the subject's judgment, and the difference between the value of the valid and invalid cue, represents a measure of response to both cues, $(V-S)/(V-I)$. By referring to the figure, one can see that as the value of the judg-

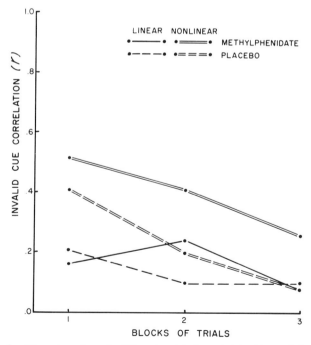

**Figure 5.4.**    Invalid cue dependency for 60 learning trials for methylphenidate and placebo groups.

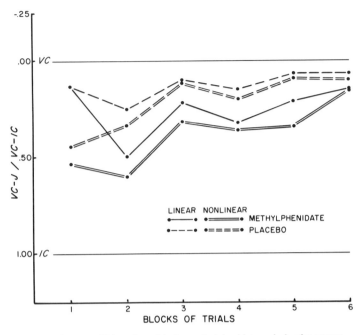

**Figure 5.5.**   Learning over 60 learning trials for methylphenidate and placebo groups.

ment approaches the value of the valid cue, the term goes to zero, indicating asymptotically perfect performance for the learning session.

### Changes in Mood

Figure 5.6 presents the results of the administrations of the MAACL. Overall premedication means for the entire sample ($n = 28$) on the three subscales were anxiety, depression, and hostility. Standardization means for 100 job applicants (JA) cited in the MAACL Manual are substantially lower (lesser symptomatology) than the subject sample on the anxiety and depression scales, and about the same on the hostility scale. Post medication scores for each subject were the average of the two scores obtained on day 4 and day 5 of medication. One-way ANOVA's were performed on the difference scores for the three subscales. On the anxiety scale, improvement in the placebo, but not the methylphenidate group is reflected in the marginally significant difference. No significant difference occurred on the depression or hostility measures. In short, administration of methylphenidate for the period of time to this subject population resulted in no significant self-reported change in mood.

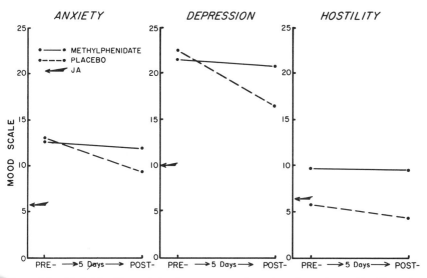

**Figure 5.6.** Methylphenidate and placebo group means for anxiety, depression, and hostility scales on the MAACL. (JA refers to standardization means representing 100 job applicants.)

## DISCUSSION

Since previous findings with amphetamine suggested facilitation of attention, concentration, and learning, it was expected that it would also enhance subjects' performance in judgmental learning tasks. Drug-induced differences in cognitive functioning did appear on the learning task but in a direction contrary to expectations. Analysis of learning in the first 60 trials showed that the placebo group learned more rapidly to utilize both cues correctly, and reached a higher asymptote, than did the methylphenidate group. Since methylphenidate is a stimulant purported to increase attentiveness and concentration, one might have expected more efficient learning, whereas the opposite result occurred. Results from the learning measure pinpointed the area of dysfunction in the methylphenidate subjects: learning to reduce dependency on the invalid cue. This evidence had appeared in trends in the invalid cue analysis as well as the consistency measure, but could be seen most clearly in the measure of learning behavior (Figure 5.5).

Not only was learning under methylphenidate impaired (contrary to expectation), but also the lack of effect of methylphenidate upon mood in the patient sample was unanticipated, particularly since the admitting diagnosis of mild depression was confirmed by the preexperimental scores on the MAACL. After 5 days of medication the only change in mood detected on the scale was a slight improvement in the placebo group on the anxiety measure, a result possibly due to several factors. Five days of medication may not have been sufficient to establish a positive change in mood, or the dosage (10 mg, t.i.d.) may not have been high enough. Although the stimulant methylphenidate is recommended for mild depression (Physician's Desk Reference, 1972), it may not be the drug of choice for this particular patient sample, some of whom had been alcoholic and therefore users of a depressant drug.

The studies reviewed at the beginning of the chapter suggest that the effect of stimulants upon intellectual functioning is to facilitate attention, arousal, and mood, but those studies used normal adult subjects or hyperkinetic children. Impairment of learning, accompanied by lack of reported improvement in mood, in mildly depressed adult males suggests that stimulants may not be useful for purposes of clinical or intellectual facilitation.

If one looks at the specific nature of the dysfunction of the methylphenidate group, however, a plausible post hoc hypothesis suggests itself. Methylphenidate, in fact, can be expected to "open" subjects to information, to increase attention and increase the effective utilization of cues. Being "open" to a range of cues is not always an adaptive cognitive framework, however, as Gillis and Davis (1973) have argued. A wide or narrow focus may have increased or decreased learning, depending on the structure of the task. The tasks used here involved subjects learning to depend on a single cue and largely to ignore the other, ecologically less valid, cue. By increasing the propensity of a subject to take account of cues, methylphenidate may have induced a cognitive state directly opposite to that which would have facilitated performance on a narrow-focus task. The invalid cue dependency maintained by methylphenidate subjects indicates that methylphenidate did result in widening of the focus of the subjects. (See Chapter 4 for a further discussion of this point.)

According to this hypothesis, the impairment of functioning by methylphenidate in a narrow-focus task is, therefore, not surprising. This drug might be expected to enhance performance where the cognitive state it induced was appropriate to the task, such as a wide-focus task requiring attention to a range of cues for successful performance. Future research that accounts for these differential task structures may find that methylphenidate is indeed an effective facilitator of learning and judgmental performance in certain contexts.

## REFERENCES

Callaway, E. The influence of amobarbital (amylobarbitone) and methamphetamine on the focus of attention. *Journal of Mental Science*, 1959, **105**, 382–392.

Conners, C. K., Eisenberg, L., and Sharpe, L. Effects of methylphenidate (Ritalin) on paired-associate learning and Porteus Maze performance in emotionally disturbed children. *Journal of Consulting Psychology*, 1964, **28**, 14–22.

Esplin, D. W. and Zablocka-Esplin, B. Central nervous system stimulants. In L. S. Goodman and A. Gilman (Eds.), *The pharmacological basis of therapeutics*. New York: Macmillan, 1970.

Gillis, J. A. and Davis, K. E. The effects of psychoactive drugs on complex thinking in paranoid and nonparanoid schizophrenics: An application of the multiple-cue model to the study of disordered thinking. In L. Rappoport and D. Summers (Eds.), *Human judgment and social interaction*. New York: Holt, Rinehart & Winston, 1973.

Herrington, R. N. The effect of amphetamine on a serial reaction task. *Psychopharmacologia*, 1967, **12**, 50–57.

Martin, W. R., Sloan, J. W., Sapira, J. D., and Jasinski, D. R. Physiologic, subjective, and behavioral effects of amphetamine, methamphetamine, ephedrine, phenmetrazine, and methylphenidate in man. *Clinical Pharmacology and Therapeutics*, 1971, **12**, 245–258.

*Physician's Desk Reference*. Medical Economics, Inc., 1972.

Quarton, G. C. and Talland, G. A. The effects of methamphetamine and pentobarbital on two measures of attention. *Psychopharmacologia*, 1962, **3**, 66–71.

Sykes, D. H., Douglas, V. I., and Morgenstern, G. The effect of methylphenidate (Ritalin) on sustained attention in hyperactive children. *Psychopharmacologia*, 1972, **25**, 262–274.

Talland, G. A. and Quarton, G. C. The effects of methamphetamine and pentobarbital on the running memory span. *Psychopharmacologia*, 1965, **7**, 379–382.

Talland, G. A. and Quarton, G. C. The effects of drugs and familiarity on performance in continuous visual search. *Journal of Nervous and Mental Disease*, 1966, **143**, 87–91.

Weiss, B. and Laties, V. G. Enhancement of human performance by caffeine and the amphetamines. *Pharmacological Reviews*, 1962, **14**, 1–36.

Weiss, G., Minde, K., Douglas, V., Werry, J., and Sykes, D. Comparison of the effects of chlorpromazine, dextroamphetamine, and methylphenidate on the behavior and intellectual functioning of hyperactive children. *Canadian Medical Association Journal*, 1971, **104**, 20–25.

Zuckerman, M. and Lubin, B. *Manual for the Multiple Affect Adjective Checklist*. San Diego: Educational and Industrial Testing Service, 1965.

(DMT), methylendioxyamphetamine (MDA), 2,5-dimethoxy-4-methyl-amphetamine (STP), phencyclidine (Sernyl), tetrahydrocannabinol (THC), morning glory seeds, and baby wood rose seeds. Marijuana and hashish were also included in this category, although they lack the potent consciousness-altering qualities of the other hallucinogens.

## PROCEDURE

### Subjects

Eighty subjects between the ages of 15 and 30 years comprised the total study sample. The sample was divided into three groups on the basis of reported drug usage: (a) frequent hallucinogenic drug users; (b) infrequent hallucinogenic drug users; and (c) nonusers of hallucinogens. In order to be included in either hallucinogenic drug user group, subjects had to have reported ingesting an hallucinogen at least once within the last four months, but not within 48 hours prior to the experimental situation.

### Frequent Hallucinogenic Drug Users

Persons who reported using hallucinogens a total of more than 50 times were assigned to the frequent hallucinogenic drug user group. Within the frequent drug user group, a total approximated hallucinogenic usage range of 56–658 ingestions, with a median of 122 ingestions, was reported. LSD-25 was the most frequently used hallucinogen. Frequent drug users used more amphetamines, opiates, stimulants, and barbiturates, as well as hallucinogens, than did the infrequent drug user group (see Table 6.1)

### Infrequent Hallucinogenic Drug Users

Persons who reported using hallucinogens a total of less than 50 times were assigned to the infrequent hallucinogenic drug user group. A range of 5–48 ingestions, with a median of 19.5 ingestions, was reported by this group.

Since the focus of the study was on long-term rather than acute effects of hallucinogens, a 48-hour drug free limit (including cannabis products) was initially imposed to decrease data contamination from acute drug effects; this limit was later decreased to 24 hours because of the scarcity of subjects, and the data was then analyzed for differential effects of the recency of marijuana usage.

Certain other guides were used to minimize the effects of other drugs that might

Table 6.1. "Street Drugs" Used by Infrequent and Frequent Drug Users: Total "Hits"/Subject—Ranges and Medians

| Type of Drug | Infrequent Users | | | Frequent Users | | |
|---|---|---|---|---|---|---|
| | Subjects | Range | Median | Subjects | Range | Median |
| Total hallucinogen usage (excluding cannabis) | 20 | 5–48 | 19.5 | 20 | 56–658 | 122 |
| Peyote | 20 | 0–4 | 0.5 | 20 | 0–10 | 2 |
| Psilocybin | 20 | 0–4 | 1 | 20 | 0–50 | 2 |
| Morning Glory Seeds | 0 | 0 | 0 | 20 | 0–3 | 0 |
| Baby Wood Rose Seeds | 20 | 0–2 | 0 | 16 | 0–20 | 0.5 |
| LSD-25 | 20 | 1–25 | 10 | 20 | 15–300 | 87.5 |
| Other hallucinogens (DET, DMT, MDA, THC, STP, & Mescaline) | 20 | 0–28 | 4.5 | 20 | 12–353 | 35 |
| Amphetamines | 20 | 0–55 | 0 | 20 | 5–1825 | 31 |
| Narcotics (Opium, Heroin, Cocaine) | 20 | 0–10 | 0 | 20 | 0–102 | 5 |
| Glue | 0 | 0 | 0 | 3 | 5–50 | |
| Quaalude | 20 | 0–10 | 0 | 20 | 0–33 | 1.5 |
| Barbiturates | 20 | 0–1 | 0 | 20 | 0–192 | 1.5 |
| Cocaine | 8 | 0–6 | | 17 | 0–40 | |

also influence cognitive processes.* Persons were excluded from the drug user samples if they had sniffed glue, gasoline, or aerosol substances more than a total of five times; if they were or ever had been physically dependent on narcotics or alcohol (as assessed by questioning if they had experienced runny noses, backaches, nausea, vomiting, blackouts, tremors, seizures, delirium tremens, etc.); if they had used more than one barbiturate or tranquilizer per day for the three months prior to participation in the study; if they had used amphetamines or other stimulants more than 35 times orally, or intravenously, or within the six months prior to participation in the study. (Two persons who exceeded the glue limitation and 11 persons who exceeded the 35 amphetamine ingestion limit were included, however, owing to the scarcity of subjects.) Persons were also excluded from the drug user sample if they reported a history of psychiatric hospitalizations to minimize the number of persons with gross psychopathology and possible functional thought disorders.

*Based on recommendations by Dr. Thomas Crowley, Department of Psychiatry, Colorado General Hospital.

*Nonhallucinogenic Drug Users (Control Group)*

Forty subjects were classified as nonhallucinogenic drug users because they reported *(a)* never having ingested any major hallucinogenic drugs; *(b)* never having smoked marijuana or smoking it less than 10 times in their lifetime, and not within the five months prior to the experiment; *(c)* not having ingested barbiturates, narcotics, tranquilizers, or stimulants within the five months prior to the study, and previously, only by medical prescription; *(d)* never having been addicted to alcohol, and *(e)* no history of psychiatric hospitalization. These criteria were also selected by the investigator upon considering research indications that chronic marijuana users required at least three months of drug abstinence before returning to a predrug level of functioning (Kolansky and Moore, 1972).

The mean age of the frequent hallucinogenic drug users was 21.1 years (range 18–26 years), and the mean educational level was 13.5 years (range 11–16 years). The mean number of years of experimentation with hallucinogens was 4.7 years (range 2–9 years). There were 5 females and 15 males in this group.

Infrequent hallucinogenic drug users had an age range of 16–29 years with a mean age of 23.4 years, and a mean educational level of 15.9 years (range 9–22 years). The mean number of years of experimentation with hallucinogens was 3.6 years (range 2–9 years). This subsample contained 6 females and 14 males.

Nonhallucinogenic drug users had an age range of 16–30 years, with a mean of 25.5 years. The mean educational level for the group was 15 years (range 10–18 years). There were 19 females and 21 males in the control group. Subjects came from five geographical locations—two cities in Colorado, two cities in Kansas, and one city in Missouri.

Because of the legal dangers of hallucinogenic drug use, four approaches were used to obtain subjects for the sample. Seven subjects responded to advertisements placed on college campuses; 41 subjects were obtained as a result of the investigator's personal search among friends, and referrals from acquaintances; subjects themselves referred an additional 14 persons; and 24 persons were obtained in response to the investigator's approaches on the street.

If a subject agreed to participate, a drug history questionnaire was administered by the investigator to ascertain the type and frequency of drugs ingested, the approximate dates on which the drugs were last used, and the route of administration. Included in the questionnaire were lists of "psychedelic drugs," narcotics, common pain killers (such as aspirin and Darvon), nonprescription sleeping pills, prescription antianxiety compounds (such as chlordiazepoxide and diazepam), barbiturates, nonbarbiturate sedative-hypnotics (such as chloral hydrate and methaqualone), major tranquilizers (such as chlorpromazine), stimulants, and diet pills. In an attempt to have subjects estimate their drug use as carefully as possible, the investigator had subjects estimate the total number of hallucinogens ingested in their lifetime and then compare this number with their reported estimates of individual hallucinogens used. Any discrepancies in estimates were then re-evaluated by the subject. Questions were also included to ascertain the subjects' alcohol consumption patterns.

Based upon the information obtained on the drug history, the individual was assigned to one of the three subject groups described above. Within the groups, subjects were alternately assigned to either the narrow-focus or the wide-focus judgmental learning task. A urine sample was collected after the hallucinogenic drug user subjects had completed the judgmental learning task. A debriefing session concluded the experimental procedure. All subjects received payment for their participation.

Urine specimens were obtained from 32 (80%) of the hallucinogenic drug user subjects who participated in the study as a check on their credibility. Urine specimens were not collected on the remaining eight subjects who were tested in Kansas and Missouri because of unavailability of laboratory facilities necessary for analysis. The urinalysis procedure used for this study was designed to detect the presence of barbiturates, cocaine, methadone, morphine, quinine, amphetamines, codeine, and unknown substances. None of the subjects included in the study sample gave urine specimens that were incompatible with their histories.

*Attrition*

Thirty-two persons approached on the street refused to participate; 2 of those persons cited a fear of being apprehended by police, 1 person refused because of lack of time, 1 person refused because he was having emotional problems, and 28 persons cited not having ingested hallucinogens in the last four months as reasons for refusal to participate. Six persons agreed to participate but failed to keep their appointments.

Eighty-six persons participated in this study, but six persons were excluded from the sample. One person was excluded because of a history of narcotic addiction, and two persons were excluded because they admitted to having smoked marijuana just prior to the time of being tested. Data from two persons were deleted from the final analysis because of histories of psychiatric hospitalizations. Data from one other person were omitted due to an inconsistency between the drug history obtained from the person and the urinalysis.

**Tasks**

As indicated, narrow-focus and wide-focus tasks were used. Each task was constructed so that uncertain relationships existed between three cues and criterion variable. For both tasks, the three cues were labeled as follows: (1) "interest in patient"; (2) "intelligence"; and (3) "age/experience." The criterion variable—the variable to be predicted from different values of the three cues —was described as "the quality of medical care received from a physician." The subject was to learn to make this prediction on the basis of differing values of the three cues observed over a series of 60 trials. The correct answer was provided after each trial.

Each task consisted of a set of 60 stimulus cards on which the three cues were displayed in graphic form on a numerical scale from 1 to 100. The criterion variable was indicated on a scale from 1 to 20. Adequate performance on the tasks required learning to detect the differential importance of the three cues in making judgments about the criterion variable.

Task *A* represented the narrow-focus task, in which nearly all of the variance was assigned to one cue ("interest in patient") with the remaining cues ("intelligence" and "age/experience") having approximately zero correlation with the criterion variable. Adequate performance on this task depended upon learning to detect the high validity of a single cue, namely, "interest in patient," and to make use of that cue in predicting the criterion variable, "quality of medical care to be received."

Task *B* represented the wide-focus task in which the total variance was distributed almost equally among the three cues. This task required that the subject learn to detect the validity of all three cues, and to make use of them, in order to achieve high performance levels. (See Figure 6.1 for a description of the statistical properties of both tasks.)

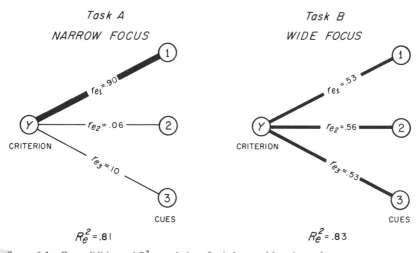

**igure 6.1**    Cue validities and $R_e^2$ correlations for judgmental learning tasks.

All subjects worked individually. The investigator explained the task instructions, and then presented the stimulus cards one at a time to the subject. Subjects were told to use the cues on the stimulus card to make judgments about the quality of medical care received from a physician. The subject then predicted a value from 1 to 20 for the criterion variable. The subject's judgments were recorded; immediate outcome feedback was given on each trial. Sixty trials were presented to each subject.

Each subject's performance was evaluated in terms of three measures: *(a)* the measure of total achievement $r_a$ attained by correlating his responses over a series of trials with the correct values of the criterion variable; *(b)* the measure of knowledge $G$ attained by calculating the relation between the subject's cue weighting system with the cue weighting system in the task; and *(c)* the measure of linear consistency $R^2$ attained by calculating the multiple correlation between the cue values and the subject's judgments. (See Hammond, Chapter 3, for further details concerning these measures.)

## RESULTS

### Effect of Frequency of Drug Use

Analysis of variance with respect to the effect of frequency of drug use revealed no statistical difference between drug user and nondrug user groups on the three performance measures described above. In general, all three groups tended to perform slightly better on the wide-focus Task $B$ than on the narrow-focus Task $A$. Although there were no statistically significant differences in performance among the three groups, infrequent drug users performed slightly better than the frequent drug user and nondrug user groups on both tasks ($F = 1.53; df = 2, 54; p > .05$).

### Effects of Recency of Marijuana Usage On Performance

The data were also examined in order to evaluate the effects of recent use of marijuana on subject performance. Table 6.2 describes the recency of usage and the numbers of subjects involved in each group. As shown in Figure 6.2, subjects who had smoked marijuana within the 48 hours just prior to their completion of the tasks performed less well than subjects who *had not* smoked marijuana within the 48 hours just prior to their completion of the tasks. Although these results were not statistically significant ($F = 0.39; df = 2, 76; p > .05$), they suggested a need to examine the possibility of *differential effects* of marijuana smoking on the two drug-user groups.

Table 6.2.    Numbers of Subjects within Groups: Use of Marijuana and Hashish

|  | Nonusers | Infrequent Users | Frequent Users |
|---|---|---|---|
| Never tried marijuana | 27 | | |
| Tried marijuana less than ten times in lifetime | 13 | | |
| Infrequent marijuana users (less than 5 "joints"/week) | | 11 | 4 |
| Daily marijuana users | | 9 | 16 |
| Smoked marijuana less than 48 hours before study | | 5 | 4 |
| Smoked marijuana more than 48 hours before study | | 15 | 16 |

This hypothesis was tested by means of a 2 (Groups: frequent versus infrequent drug users) × 2 (Conditions: using marijuana more than 48 hours prior to participation versus less than 48 hours prior to participation) × 3 (Blocks) analysis of variance with repeated measurements on the third factor. (Tasks were not included as a factor because of the small $n$ within one or more cells.) A measure of overall achievement $r_a$ showed a clear interaction between Groups × Conditions ($F = 4.52$; $df = 1, 36$; $p < .05$).

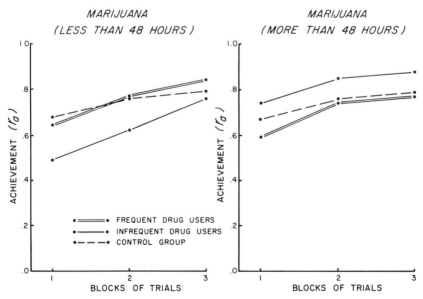

Figure 6.2.    Achievement $r_a$ correlations: interaction between frequency of hallucinogenic drug use and time of marijuana drug use prior to testing.

As may be seen from Figure 6.2, the effects of prior smoking of marijuana are such that the overall performance of the frequent drug users was *enhanced*, while the overall performance of the infrequent drug users was *impaired*. Investigation of the question of whether the disparity in learning between these groups was due to the differential acquisition of knowledge $G$ or to difference in control $R^2$, shows that the difference was clearly due to control $R^2$ (see Figures 6.3 and 6.4). There were no statistically significant differences in $G$, whereas there was a statistically significant interaction (similar to that obtained for $r_a$) in $R^2$.

The decrement due to absence of marijuana observed in the performance of the frequent drug users was, therefore, caused by their inability to execute their judgments *consistently*, rather than to an inability to ascertain the properties of the tasks accurately. The effect of marijuana use on infrequent drug users, on the other hand, was to induce a loss of such cognitive control. In neither case, however, were the subjects' abilities to acquire knowledge about the task affected by the use or absence of use of marijuana in the 48 hours preceding participation in the study.

It should also be noted that whereas the differences between all three groups were marginal, the frequent drug users who had recently smoked marijuana

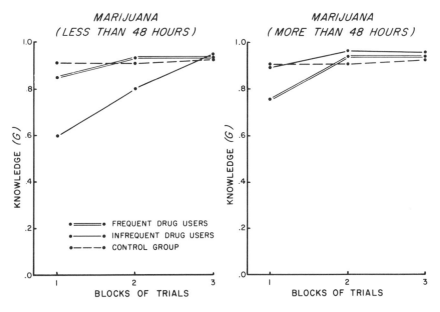

**Figure 6.3.** Knowledge $G$ correlations: interaction between frequency of hallucinogenic drug use and time of marijuana drug use prior to testing.

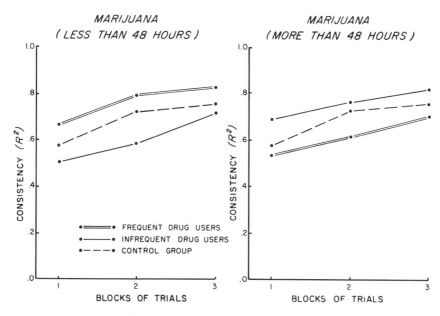

**Figure 6.4.**    Consistency $R$ ${}^2_s$ correlations: interaction between frequency of hallucinogenic drug use and time of marijuana drug use prior to testing.

performed *better* than the control subjects (primarily because of better cognitive control, higher $R^2$'s; see Figure 6.4). Similarly, the infrequent users who had recently smoked marijuana performed less well than the controls (again because of a difference in cognitive control). If this result were confirmed, it would carry considerable significance, for it would indicate a factual basis for the as yet unconfirmed and conflicting reports by drug users of "street drugs" of improved performance after smoking marijuana.

The results of this study suggest that hallucinogenic drug users were able to learn to improve their judgment in two different probabilistic judgment tasks, and that their performance did not differ from that of control subjects. The recent use of marijuana prior to task performance, however, *enhanced* the performance of the frequent drug users, although it *impaired* the performance of the infrequent drug users. The specific effect of marijuana was to increase the control frequent drug users exercised over their judgments, but to decrease the control infrequent drug users exercised over their judgments. There were no statistically significant differences between groups with regard to acquisition of knowledge about the tasks.

## DISCUSSION

The unknown quality and quantity of the drugs reported used by the subjects make it impossible to draw conclusions about specific pharmacological agents, of course. As is commonly known, "street drugs" frequently are sold as mescaline or THC when, in fact, they are another agent, such as LSD, Sernyl or a mixture of agents. Although a few of the drug user subjects occasionally had their street drugs analyzed at free clinics, most of the drug users in the present study acknowledged during the interview that they really did not know the types and amounts of drugs they had ingested. Therefore, the conclusions to be drawn from the present study must be related to the effects on cognitive performance of a large conglomerate of materials bought and sold without reliable information as to either substance or quantity.

The significance of the results lies in their social-psychological implications: namely, how habitual use of "street drugs" affects the judgmental learning capabilities of persons who use them, and how the use of marijuana affects frequent and infrequent "street drug" users. Although pure cause-effect knowledge of specific hallucinogenic drugs, such as LSD, is useful, very few persons use such drugs in their pure form. And just as the results of the present study cannot be applied to the laboratory situation, neither can results of laboratory studies be generalized to the "street." Each type of study has its own purpose.

The present study offers information about hallucinogenic drug users that, if supported by further research, suggests a social cause of habituation. For example, if a frequent drug user functions better within his environment after using marijuana and less well if he has not used marijuana for 48 hours, then improvement after smoking marijuana might serve as a reinforcement for continuing to smoke marijuana frequently. An infrequent drug user, however, performs better if he has not smoked marijuana for 48 hours. Therefore, marijuana is a negative reinforcer for infrequent drug users. As is well known (Krasner, 1958; Atthowe & Krasner, 1968; O'Leary & Becker, 1967), negative reinforcers tend to be less potent than positive reinforcers; therefore, impairment due to marijuana smoking would not be expected to deter the infrequent user very much, if he were also receiving large amounts of social reinforcement from his peers for smoking marijuana. If social reinforcement does increase the use of hallucinogens for a given person, the same drug (marijuana) which was formerly a negative reinforcer in cognitive task situations will now become a positive reinforcer. The use of both hallucinogens and marijuana would thus become cumulatively greater. Further research on the use of "street drugs" is, of course, necessary to substantiate this speculation.

# REFERENCES

Atthowe, J. M., Jr., and Krasner, L. Preliminary report on the application of contingent reinforcement procedures (token economy) on a "chronic" psychiatric ward. *Journal of Abnormal Psychology*, 1968, **73**, 37–43.

Blacker, K., Jones, R., Stone, G., and Pfefferbaum, D. Chronic users of LSD. *American Journal of Psychiatry*, 1968, **125**, 341–351.

Cohen, S. and Edwards, A. E. LSD and organic brain damage. *Drug Dependence*, 1969, **2**, 118–127.

Kolansky, H. and Moore, W. T. Toxic effects of chronic marijuana use. *Journal of the American Medical Association*, 1972, **222**, 35–41.

Krasner, L. Studies of the conditioning of verbal behavior. *Psychological Bulletin*, 1958, **55**, 148–170.

McGlothlin, W., Arnold, D., and Freedman, D. Organicity measures following repeated LSD ingestion. *Archives of General Psychiatry*, 1969, **21**, 704–709.

O'Leary, K. D. and Becker, W. C. Behavior modification of an adjustment class: A token reinforcement program. *Exceptional Children*, 1967, **33**, 637–642.

CHAPTER 7

# Effects of Chlorpromazine and Thiothixene on Acute Schizophrenic Patients

JOHN S. GILLIS

Considerable research has been directed to the study of conflicting judgments (see Chapter 3) and how individuals resolve them. In particular, this research has been concerned with determining the methods by which persons resolve their differences, the limits of such attempts at resolution and, most important, the conditions likely to facilitate or impede effective reduction of conflict.

In order to assess these critical aspects of conflict resolution, Hammond (1965) has developed an experimental paradigm based on Brunswik's "lens model" (Brunswik, 1955, 1956), described in detail in Chapter 3. The research paradigm (a) brings together persons having differing judgmental systems, and (b) confronts such persons with problems admitting no perfect solution. The first condition is obviously necessary if conflict is to occur, and the second is justified on the grounds that issues about which individuals hold different policies or beliefs are seldom susceptible to perfect solution. The social judgment theory conflict paradigm not only allows the fulfillment of these conditions but enables the experimenter to design tasks that create cognitive differences between subjects; both the nature and magnitude of disagreement are under experimental control.

Since the initial investigations by Rappoport (1965) and Hammond (1965), there have been a number of conflict studies that explored the differences and similarities in the manner of dealing with such disagreements among various national groups. There are basic similarities in the way in which individuals from a variety of backgrounds resolve their differences (see Chapter 3). Most important, the research results suggest that conflict resolution is exceedingly slow and has definite (and predictable) limits. Moreover, the results indicate that as interactions ("negotiations") between the parties continue, subjects become increasingly inconsistent in their policies, thereby making compromise difficult. The effects of psychoactive drugs on the resolution of cognitive conflict is a problem that certainly deserves attention. Since the reduction of interpersonal conflict is partially a function of learning (learning *from* another about the task; learning *about* the other person's reasons for his decisions), one might expect psychoactive drugs to exert some influence on conflict simply because they effect learning. The possible differential effects of psychoactive drugs on such parameters of judgmental performance as knowledge and cognitive control (considered in Chapter 3) are also directly relevant to the study of conflict resolution.

The present study is concerned with the effects of selected antipsychotic drugs on the process and limits of conflict reduction. The data reported here were obtained as part of a larger study of the effects of antipsychotic drugs on a variety of objective and interpersonal judgment indices. Some details of the whole experiment have already been considered in Chapter 4 , and the reader will be referred to that chapter for such information.

## METHOD

Details of method, drugs evaluated, and characteristics of the sample are described in Chapter 4. The drugs used were chlorpromazine (CPZ; Thorazine) and thiothixene (Navane); the sample consisted of hospitalized adolescent acute schizophrenics.

### Tasks

The conflict model (the triple-system case) and its general implementation are considered in detail in Chapter 3. The specific types of tasks and procedures used with the schizophrenic subjects are described here.

The conflict paradigm has two stages: (1) a learning stage in which subjects learn to use information in different ways, and (2) an interactive or conflict stage in which subjects with differential learning are brought together to solve problems jointly. The interpersonal learning (IPL) stage is added to this conflict procedure so that subjects having worked together on problems in the interactive phase are now required, for a designated series of trials, to give not only their own response to the problem, but also to predict, on the basis of their interactions with him, their partner's response.

In this study, subjects learned to judge the quality of "teachers" based on two items of information: *(a)* how intelligent the teacher was and *(b)* how much discipline he maintained in the classroom. The tasks were not capable of perfect solution at either the learning or interactive stages. Predictability was high, however, $R^2$ (the squared multiple correlation between the cues and the criterion) was .98 for both the learning and interactive trials.

## Learning Stage

Stimulus materials for the learning stage consisted of 60 cards, each representing a different teacher. Two scales (vertical bars as used in the social judgment tasks) were depicted on each card: (1) one scale giving information regarding the intelligence of the teacher; and (2) the other scale designating the level of discipline he maintained in the classroom. Both were 10-point scales, the level of each variable represented by the height of a black bar. Subjects were thus provided with precise indices of the two variables relevant to the judgments they were to make. The criterion they were attempting to predict, "quality of teacher," ranged from 1 to 20; higher scores being associated with the better teachers.

Two sets of learning stimuli were used: (1) one in which virtually all of the variance in the criterion was attributable to the "intelligence" variable, the correlation between "discipline" and "quality of teacher" being essentially zero; and (2) one in which this cue-criterion relationship was reversed, that is, variance in the criterion was accounted for by the "discipline" cue, the correlation between "intelligence" and "quality" being zero. The training tasks were further differentiated in that the cue-criterion relationship was linear in one of these (intelligence and quality), while "discipline" related to teacher quality in a curvilinear fashion. Both extremes, too much and too little discipline, were associated with low values of the criterion.

Subjects to be paired in the second (conflict) and third (IPL) stages of the study were randomly assigned to one of these two learning conditions.

## Interactive Stage

In this second stage of the study subjects who had learned to use different cues (either "intelligence" or "discipline") were paired to make joint decisions. Each pair contained one member who was receiving medication according to one of the three experimental treatment regimens (chlorpromazine, thiothixene, or placebo) and a partner selected from among available patients in a ward for acutely disturbed adolescents.

This interactive stage consisted of 20 trials. Subjects were told that, as before, they would be making decisions about the quality of teachers based on knowledge of their intelligence and discipline in the classroom, but would now also be required to reach a jointly acceptable prediction as well as individual decisions. They were not informed that they had learned different tasks, or that the cue validities were different from those in the learning task. During this interactive stage both cues had the same validity ($r = .67$). A compromise between judgments derived from the learning tasks was thus required for maximally accurate joint decisions.

### Reinforcement for Performance

At this point financial incentives for performance were introduced. Motivation —or more correctly, lack of it—has traditionally been recognized as a basic symptom of schizophrenia and a major drawback to research with these patients. In order to enhance motivation in these reasonably complex and demanding interactive tasks, each subject was given 25 cents for every trial of the 20 interactive trials, in which the *joint* response was within ± 2 of the correct answer. It was therefore possible for each subject to earn as much as $5.00 in this second stage of the experiment.

## RESULTS AND DISCUSSION

The important measures in research on cognitive conflict are those relating to agreement, knowledge, and consistency. The drugs selected were compared with respect to the degree to which subjects were able to achieve agreement, and on the consistency they were able to maintain when confronted with altered task demands as well as a partner having a different judgment policy.

### Agreement

The most direct way of examining the reduction of differences between pairs of subjects is by correlating their judgments over trials. The average correlations $r_A$ (z-transformations) across all pairs in a given treatment condition were determined. This analysis was separately accomplished for both the first and the second blocks of 10 trials in the interactive stage. The results are plotted for each of the three treatment groups in Figure 7.1.

As can be seen in Figure 7.1, the placebo group is the first to begin to resolve their differences. Although the thiothixene subjects began to eliminate differences later—the correlation among subjects' responses in the first block of trials is approximately .0 —they are attaining the same level of agreement as placebo subjects by the second block of interaction trials. Perhaps the most remarkable

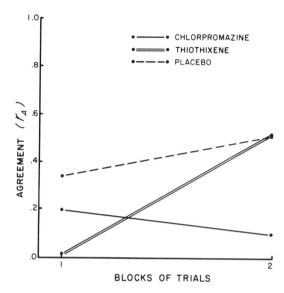

**Figure 7.1.** Agreement $r_A$ under three drug conditions.

result is that chlorpromazine subjects are significantly inferior to both placebo and thiothixene subjects in resolving differences at the completion of the joint interaction trials ($t = 2.10$; $df = 17$; $p = .05$). The implications of this important result, indicating that chlorpromazine makes it difficult to learn *from* another person are considered below.

## Knowledge

Hammond and Summers (1972) have noted the importance of analyzing achievement according to its knowledge and control components. The index of knowledge G is described in detail by Hammond (Chapter 3). The results for this index are summarized for each drug group over two blocks of trials in Figure 7.2. As described there, placebo subjects learn to use cues in a manner similar to their partner in the *first* block of trials. During the *second* block, both placebo and thiothixene subjects achieve similarity in cue utilization with their partners.

The most striking aspect of these results is, however, the markedly inferior performance of chlorpromazine subjects in block 2. These subjects actually deteriorate; they use cue information in a way *decreasingly* similar to their partners as interaction continues. These results are, of course, congruent with the findings concerning agreement reported above.

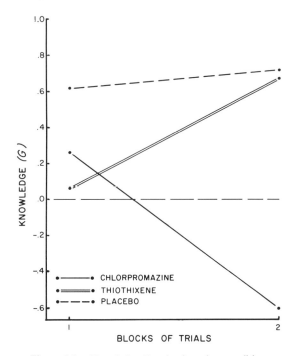

**Figure 7.2.**    Knowledge $G$ under three drug conditions.


*Consistency*

The measure of consistency employed for the interactive task was $R^2$, the squared multiple correlation between the values of the cues available (in this case the two cues relating to intelligence and discipline) and a subject's responses. It was expected that subjects who learned a linear or nonlinear cue might be differentially consistent (see also Chapter 3). The $R^2$ for each group was therefore separately assessed for both the first and second block of trials. The results are described for the three treatment groups in Figures 7.3 and 7.4.

Of the subjects who learned the linear cue (intelligence), the order of consistency of policy is identical with that obtained for the narrow-focus learning task (Chapter 4). That is, placebo subjects are most consistent, with thiothixene subjects next, and the chlorpromazine subjects significantly below both of these. For subjects who learned the nonlinear cue, drug condition seems to make less difference (Figure 7.4) although the placebo group is still somewhat more consistent than either of the drug groups.

Given the disruptive effects of chlorpromazine and thiothixene on learning

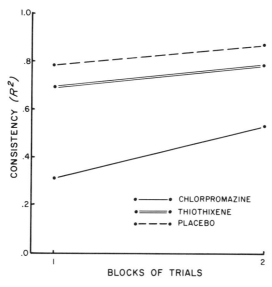

**Figure 7.3.** Consistency $R^2$ of linear subjects under three drug conditions.

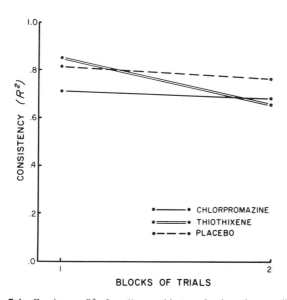

**Figure 7.4.** Consistency $R^2$ of nonlinear subjects under three drug conditions.

cue-criterion relationships in an objective task (Chapter 4), it might be expected that subjects receiving such drugs would also have difficulty learning (1) altered cue-criterion relationships and (2) the cue-criterion dependencies of another person. In the interaction stage of the experiment such learning is precisely what was required. Subjects were confronted with cue-criterion patterns for which their prior learning was inappropriate *and* they had to deal with (and resolve differences with) another individual employing a policy opposed to their own.

As Figures 7.1 to 7.4 indicate, the drugs have a disruptive effect similar to that observed on the judgmental tasks. Placebo subjects resolve their differences sooner and ultimately much more effectively than do chlorpromazine patients (Figures 7.1 and 7.2) and are more consistent in their approach to problems than either drug group (Figures 7.3 and 7.4). The diminished consistency of the drug subjects suggests that their inability to resolve differences derives from their more erratic approach to the problems. Maximally successful—and financially rewarded—performance depends here on both partners implementing their learning task policies and then compromising these individual judgments in the joint decision. Inconsistency on the part of either partner would make it difficult to effect a compromise. It is, of course, difficult to learn anything from an individual who does not have a stable approach to the problem. This is precisely what happened to patients receiving these drugs, especially in the chlorpromazine group. Finding that their previous method of dealing with the problem was ineffective, they became less stable, thus making it difficult to resolve differences with their partner. Their partner, in turn, could learn little from them because of the erratic nature of their approach.

It is useful, as Hammond and others (Hammond & Summers, 1972; Hammond, Summers, & Deane, 1973; Slovic, 1973) suggest, to think of "consistency" as reflecting the *control* aspect of cognitive behavior. The consistency measure $R^2$ does not reflect the knowledge of how information should be utilized but rather the capacity to implement effectively such knowledge (or to execute one's policy). This cognitive control function is adversely affected by the psychoactive chemicals used in this study, the results with regard to conflict resolution being congruent with those on objective task learning; the superiority of the placebo group was demonstrated in *both* the judgmental learning and interactive tasks. That cognitive control is impaired by these tranquilizing drugs is an important (and surprising) result since they have traditionally been associated with *enhanced* control of motor and emotional behaviors (Klein & Davis, 1969; Klerman, 1970).

Not only is consistency impaired with chlorpromazine however, but also knowledge—here learning to use cue information in a way similar to that of one's partner—is affected in a strikingly negative manner. Therefore these subjects actually learn to use cues in a way decreasingly similar to their partners as interactions continue. These findings suggest that chlorpromazine makes agreement with one's partner difficult because *both* components of the agreement index, knowledge and control, are impaired. Chlorpromazine renders subjects both unable to adapt a cue utilization strategy congruent with that of their partner, and unable to maintain a consistent judgmental policy of their own. Whereas the argument is developed fully at the conclusion of Chapter 10, it is clear that such effects would make the kinds of interpersonal communication and learning required in psychological therapies difficult indeed.

## REFERENCES

Brunswik, E. Representative design and probabilistic theory in a functional psychology. *Psychological Review*, 1955, **62**, 193–217.

Brunswik, E. *Perception and the representative design of experiments*. Berkeley: University of California Press, 1956.

Hammond, K. R. New directions in research on conflict resolution. *Journal of Social Issues*, 1965, **21**, 44–66.

Hammond, K. R. and Summers, D. A. Cognitive control. *Psychological Review*, 1972, **79**, 58–67.

Hammond, K. R., Summers, D. A., and Deane, D. H. Negative effects of outcome feedback in multiple-cue probability learning. *Organizational Behavior and Human Performance*, 1973, **9**, 30–34.

Klein, D. F. and Davis, J. M. *Diagnosis and drug treatment of psychiatric disorders.* Baltimore: Williams and Wilkins, 1969.

Klerman, G. L. Clinical efficacy and actions of antipsychotics. In A. DiMascio and R. Shader (Eds.), *Clinical handbook of psychopharmacology*. New York: Science House, 1970.

Rappoport, L. Interpersonal conflict in cooperative and uncertain situations. *Journal of Experimental Social Psychology*, 1965, **1**, 323–333.

Slovic, P. Policy implementation as skilled thinking. Paper presented at the Sixth Annual Conference on Human Judgment, Boulder, Colorado, 1973.

CHAPTER 8

# Effects of Methylphenidate on Mildly Depressed Hospitalized Adults

ELLEN R. GRITZ

Although the effects of stimulants on interactive behavior in humans have not been extensively studied, the problem is obviously an important one. This study addresses itself to the question of whether the administration of methylphenidate enhances or impairs the reduction of interpersonal conflict between mildly depressed patients. Since stimulants are used therapeutically for mood disturbance, psychoneuroses, and other mild mental disorders, enhancement of mental functioning was anticipated. Drug effects are, of course, patient and dose dependent; for example, high doses of amphetamine can produce "... restlessness, dizziness, tremor, hyperactive reflexes, talkativeness, tenseness, irritability, weakness, insomnia, fever, and sometimes euphoria [Innes & Nickerson, 1970, p. 504]." However, using a moderate therapeutic dose, as was done in this study, the energizing actions of methylphenidate would be expected to affect interpersonal communication positively. Since depressed patients usually interact less than normals, a mildly depressed placebo group might be less intent on finding a quick and agreeable joint decision than would a comparable group taking low-to-moderate doses of stimulants. One might logically predict enhancement of performance under a stimulant as subjects became more attentive to one another's judgments in seeking to reach a joint decision.

Differential effects of stimulants on individual and group behavior have, however, been reported. Starkweather (1959) found that individual performance on the trail-making test was facilitated in normal subjects given a single dose of $l$-amphetamine, a usual finding on simple psychomotor tasks. When two subjects were tested in a cooperative situation, however, the performance of any subject paired with a partner given $d$-amphetamine was slowed (regardless of whether that subject had received $d$-amphetamine, phenobarbital, or placebo). Such changes in performance dependent upon a partner's responding probably involve changes in self-perception of performance compared to perception of partner's performance. Using judgmental tasks similar to those employed in this book, Gillis and Davis (1973) and Davis, Evans, and Gillis (1969) found that methamphetamine enhances performance on certain tasks with both schizophrenic and normal subjects.

The studies cited above suggest that pairs of subjects receiving methylphenidate might actually be impaired compared to placebo controls, although individual behaviors are facilitated. In view of the diagnostic category of the patient sample and the dosage selected, it was hypothesized that enhancement of performance would occur under the selected experimental conditions.

## METHOD

The learning situation described in Chapter 5 served as a learning condition for the interpersonal conflict phase of the study. Within each drug condition, pairs of subjects were brought together on day 5 of medication for a joint decision session. Each member of the pair had learned to depend on a different cue and to utilize a different function form from the other. Using the same task as in learning (rating teachers), independent judgments and joint judgments were obtained, as well as a final private judgment on 20 trials (see Gillis, Chapter 7). Measures of performance included agreement $r_A$ , knowledge $G$, consistency $R^2$, and changes in valid and invalid cue dependencies.

## PROCEDURE

### Drugs

The drugs were administered as described in Chapter 5. That is, methylphenidate hydrochloride (10 mg, t.i.d.) or placebo were each administered to two groups of subjects (14 subjects per group) for 5 days.

### Task

As in nearly all of the studies in this volume, the task (see Chapters 3, 4, and 7) used in the conflict phase of the experiment was different from both of the learning tasks. Each cue correlated .49 with the criterion and contributed equally to it. The task continued to include uncertainty ($R^2 = .98$). As in the other conflict studies the subjects were presented with 20 (5 × 8) cards that contained two cues (intelligence and leniency) in the form of vertical bars; each card described a hypothetical teacher. The subjects each made an independent decision, then reached agreement on a joint judgment through discussion; finally, they recorded a private decision after this process. The experimenter provided the correct answer (outcome feedback).

## RESULTS

### Agreement $r_A$

There was significant increase in $r_A$, the amount of agreement or correlation between judgments of $S_1$ and $S_2$, from the first to the second half of the conflict phase, but there were no significant differences between the methylphenidate and placebo groups on this measure, although performance of the placebo group was superior (see Figure 8.1).

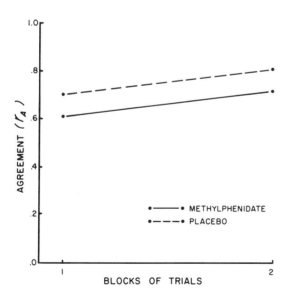

**Figure 8.1.**    Agreement $r_A$ under two drug conditions.

## Knowledge G

No differences on G, a measure of agreement corrected for inconsistency in judgment, were found between groups; this measure was already so high in the first 10 trials that no statistical improvement was evident (see Figure 8.2).

## Consistency $R^2$

The placebo group performed marginally better on $R^2$, the consistency measure (see Figure 8.3). The judgments of the subjects receiving placebo (both linear and nonlinear) became more consistent over the 20 trials, as did those of the linear methylphenidate subjects; but the nonlinear methylphenidate subjects became less consistent. The significant triple interaction Drug × Subject × Trial Block ($F$ = 5.21; $df$ = 1, 24; $p$ < .05) refers to this effect, an uneven change in the performance of the various groups during the conflict trials.

## Changes in Cue Dependency

Analysis of the cue dependency data (Figures 8.4 and 8.5) showed that linear subjects retained their dependency on their valid cue throughout the 20 trials of the

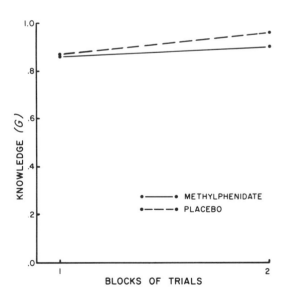

**Figure 8.2.**    Knowledge G under two drug conditions.

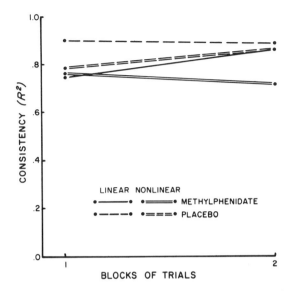

**Figure 8.3.**  Consistency $R^2$ for both linear and nonlinear subjects under two drug conditions.

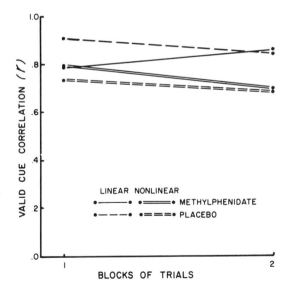

**Figure 8.4.**  Retention of dependency on the previously valid cue $r$ by linear and nonlinear subjects under two drug conditions.

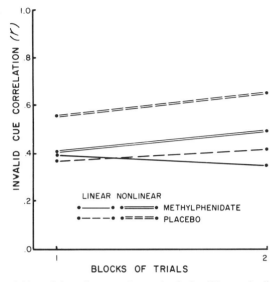

**Figure 8.5.**   Acquisition of dependency on the previously invalid cue $r$ by linear and nonlinear subjects under two drug conditions.

joint learning session more than nonlinear subjects did. The significant triple interaction indicated that the linear subjects receiving methylphenidate actually increased their dependence on their valid cue, instead of decreasing it as the other groups did ($F = 6.39$; $df = 1, 24$; $p < .05$).

Analysis of the invalid cue data showed that the nonlinear subjects in both groups developed more dependence upon the (linear) cue of the other than did the linear subjects throughout the 20 trials ($F = 4.35$; $df = 1, 24$; $p < .05$). Although the difference was not significant, the linear subjects on methylphenidate actually *decreased* their dependence on the invalid cue, instead of acquiring dependence on it. This is consistent with the finding that they wrongly increased their dependence on the valid cue at the same time.

## DISCUSSION

It was hypothesized that methylphenidate would improve performance on the conflict phase by promoting attention to, and therefore learning from, the partner and by increasing social interaction. However, methylphenidate subjects actually manifested several disturbances in cognitive functioning when compared to the placebo subjects. Nonlinear methylphenidate subjects decreased their consistency $R^2$ in the conflict phase, and linear methylphenidate subjects both increased their dependence on the cue they had learned and decreased their dependence on the cue of the other, precisely the opposite of what successful interaction calls for. Since there were no drug-induced differences in overall agreement $r_A$ or in knowledge $G$, it appears that the consistency measure $R^2$ and the change in cue dependencies were the functions impaired by methylphenidate in the conflict trials. These results support the findings in Chapter 5 of impaired learning behavior in the methylphenidate group, and poorer (although not significantly) performance on the other measures of learning (achievement, knowledge, consistency, and relinquishing of invalid cue dependency). Since all subjects were brought to the same criterion during the learning phase, the results of the conflict analysis cannot be attributed to *differences* in learning.

Evidence in the literature does point to impairing effects of stimulants upon cooperative task performance (Starkweather, 1959). The findings of this study therefore are not unprecedented. It is possible that the drug made subjects more argumentative and less willing to change their opinions. The methylphenidate linear subjects actually increased dependence on their valid cues and decreased dependence on their invalid cues, instead of modifying these dependencies in the direction of their partners' judgmental systems, although knowledge of the other's cue dependencies and overall achievement remained unimpaired.

Since the only deviations from appropriate task solution behavior were made by the methylphenidate group, it is reasonable to conclude that methylphenidate had a deleterious effect upon their cognitive abilities in a situation involving conflicting judgments.

## REFERENCES

Davis, K. E., Evans, W. O., and Gillis, J. S. The effects of amphetamine and chlorpromazine on cognitive skills and feelings in normal adult males. In W. O. Evans and N. Kline (Eds.), *The psychopharmacology of the normal human.* Springfield: Charles C. Thomas, 1969.

Gillis, J. S. and Davis, K. E. The effects of psychoactive drugs on complex thinking in paranoid and nonparanoid schizophrenics: An application of the multiple-cue model to the study of disordered thinking. In L. Rappoport and D. Summers (Eds.), *Human judgment and social interaction.* New York: Holt, Rinehart & Winston, 1973.

Innes, I. R. and Nickerson, M. Drugs acting on postganglionic adrenergic nerve endings and structures innervated by them (sympathomimetic drugs). In L. S. Goodman and A. Gillman (Eds.), *The pharmacological basis of therapeutics.* (4th ed.) New York: Macmillan, 1970.

Starkweather, J. A. Individual and situational influences on drug effects. In R. M. Featherstone and A. Simon (Eds.), *A pharmacologic approach to the study of the mind.* Springfield: Charles C. Thomas, 1959.

CHAPTER 9

# Effects of Methylphenidate and Barbiturate on Normal Subjects

N. ZACHARIADIS and D. VARONOS

This study concerns the effects of psychoactive drugs on *normal* young adults. All other studies in this book (with the exception of Chapter 12) deal with the effect of such drugs on persons whose social judgment has been called into question, and who receive psychoactive drugs in the hope that their judgment will be improved, or in one case (Zimbelman, Chapter 6), where the effects of illicit drugs used for recreational purposes are examined. The significance of the present chapter, then, lies in the question of whether normal human judgment can be improved, and thus lead to *constructive* conflict reduction in situations where judgments differ.

It is obvious that cognitive processes can be *impaired* by biochemical means, even by those drugs intended to improve judgment (see any chapter in Part II of this volume), but it has yet to be demonstrated that human judgment can be improved by biochemical means. The research paradigm used throughout this research effort presents an excellent opportunity, however, to investigate this possibility.

The specific aim of this study was to investigate the differential effects of two opposite types of drugs on the ability of young *normal* adults to reach agreement in a situation where conflict was evoked by differing judgments; the drugs employed were methylphenidate hydrochloride, pentobarbital, and a placebo. The use of a stimulant and a depressant drug also provided an opportunity to investigate further a hypothesis put forth by Gillis (Gillis & Davis, 1973; Davis, Evans, & Gillis, 1969) and Gritz (Chapters 5 and 11); see also Eysenck (1963, 1967) for a somewhat parallel view. Gillis argues that amphetamines make individuals more receptive to environmental stimuli; that is, amphetamine induces attention to and utilization of a wider range of cues in perceptual or judgmental tasks. Whether amphetamine facilitates or impairs performance is dependent on the appropriateness of this cognitive style to task characteristics. In tasks requiring attention to a wide range of cues, methylphenidate should facilitate performance. When utilization of only limited aspects of a stimulus array is necessary, methylphenidate might actually impair performance, that is, subjects would be disposed to take account of cues having low ecological validities.

The opposite cognitive consequences might be hypothesized for pentobarbital. That is, pentobarbital might be expected to narrow the range of cues to which an individual could attend and effectively utilize. Again, whether this style was adaptive or maladaptive would depend on task structure. In judgmental situations calling for the use of several cues, pentobarbital would be expected to impair performance, whereas it would facilitate functioning in tasks requiring attention to a limited number of cues.

On the basis of Gillis' reasoning, differential drug effects would be predicted in both the conflict and interpersonal learning segments. Methylphenidate would in general be expected to facilitate the reduction of conflict and enhance interpersonal learning. The resolution of conflict is enhanced if the judgment policy of another person is incorporated in one's own policy. Methylphenidate, in "opening up" the subject to the policy of the other person, should facilitate learning about the other and thereby hasten the resolution of differences. The hypotheses that follow from this reasoning include superior performance by the methylphenidate group on several conflict indices—agreement $r_A$, covert and overt conflict, and knowledge $G$.

The conflict situation also requires that subjects yield their total dependency on a single cue and take account of a cue that was not highly correlated with the criterion during learning. Again, Gillis would predict that methylphenidate should facilitate attention to an additional cue and that pentobarbital would impair it.

## METHOD

Subjects learned to use one of two cues in predicting the value of a criterion in the manner described in detail in Chapters 3 and 4. Subjects were then given tablets containing methylphenidate, pentobarbital, or placebo, and pairs of subjects who had been given the same drug participated in a series of 20 conflict trials. Results for these conflict trials are described in this chapter; results for a series of interpersonal learning trials are discussed in Chapter 12.

# PROCEDURE

## Task Materials

The materials used in this study were contentless; that is, the cues were labeled A and B, and the criterion variable was labeled C. As in the other studies described here, subjects were differentially trained to criterion, and they engaged in 20 trials in the conflict phase.

## Subjects

Ninety-six subjects (48 male and 48 female) were randomly selected according to the index number of their student cards, out of a population of 900 third-year medical students at Athens University.

## Learning

Students were invited to participate in an experiment at the Experimental Pharmacology Laboratory at Athens University. The subjects were randomly paired to form 48 same-sex pairs, each of which was instructed to call at the laboratory at 8:30 AM. Upon being seated in the laboratory room, the subject who was to learn to depend on the nonlinear cue began the task immediately. The subject who was to learn to depend on the linear cue was asked to wait for a half hour; his (or her) learning task began at 9 AM. The subject who learned to depend on the nonlinear cue was given an opportunity to start the task early because previous experience had indicated that more learning time was often required to learn to acquire the appropriate nonlinear cue dependency; it was considered essential that the tablets containing the chemical compounds be administered to both subjects at the same time. By 10 AM, all subjects had reached criterion ($r > .75$ on the cue to be depended on, $r < .25$ on the cue to be ignored, and $R_s^2 > .75$; see Chapter 3 for further detail on the procedure). No subjects were dropped from the study because of a failure to learn, or for other reasons.

## Drug Administration

At 10 AM each member of a pair received 75 mg of pentobarbital, or 10 mg of methylphenidate hydrochloride, or a placebo. Both members of a pair received the same compound. The specific contents of the capsules were unknown to the investigators and the subjects, although the investigators knew which drugs were being used. The capsules were identical in appearance. The subjects rested until 10:45 AM, in order to allow time for the drug to be absorbed. Subjects occupied themselves by reading. They were not permitted to drink coffee, tea, or other beverages affecting the central nervous system (CNS).

At 10:45 AM the subjects began the conflict phase of the study. Subjects read the directions for this phase of the experiment, and the first conflict trial was administered at approximately 11 AM.

## RESULTS

The statistically significant findings with respect to the effects of drugs were limited in this study, but there were a number of findings that did not reach traditional levels of statistical significance that are discussed in light of the predictions generated from the hypotheses discussed above.

### Effects Not Involving Drug Groups

Almost all findings that were significant at the .05 level or better involve a main effect or interaction effect for blocks of conflict trials. Improved performance during the conflict trials is demonstrated by statistically significant changes in $r_A$, $G$, $R^2$, the valid cue, the invalid cue, and cognitive change $(S - Y)$ (for the last measure the result is significant only if the placebo group is not included). These measures, as well as their importance with respect to comparable analyses, are discussed elsewhere in this book (see especially Chapter 3), and the material need not be repeated in detail here. However, results for two of the measures, the valid cue and invalid cue, are considered as illustrative of the use of the methodology described in the present volume. The discussion of these variables leads directly into a consideration of the effects of drugs.

"Valid cue" refers to dependence on the cue a subject learned to use before the interactive conflict phase of the experiment. Since this cue is *less* valid as a predictor of the criterion during conflict, the correlation, for a given subject, between values of this cue and values of the criterion should *decline* during conflict to the extent the subject's performance on the task improves.

The "invalid cue" is then the cue that was *not* valid during learning. The subject must learn to use this cue during conflict in order to adapt to the task, and the cue-criterion correlation should increase. Therefore, optimal performance on the task requires equal weighting of the valid cue and the invalid cue during conflict, and this convergence should be greatest during the second block of 10 conflict trials, as subjects learn about the task.

The valid-cue and invalid-cue correlations with the criterion were analyzed using an analysis of variance with the two 10-trial conflict blocks as a repeated measure variable; drug group, sex, and linear-cue and nonlinear-cue learning (discussed below) were "between subjects" variables. (A $z$-transformation of the correlation coefficients was done prior to analysis. Averages given below and plotted in the figures were obtained by transforming results from the analyses back to correlation coefficients.)

The effect for the two blocks of conflict trials was statistically significant at the .01 level for the analysis of the valid cue ($F = 11.06; df = 1, 60; p < .01$) and at the .05 level for the invalid-cue analysis ($F = 5.66; df = 1, 60; p < .05$). This implies that the correlation between each of these cues and the subject's judgments changed during the conflict trials and that this result was statistically reliable. The correlation between the valid cue and the judgments declined from .84 to .78 during conflict, and the invalid-cue correlation with the judgments increased from .43 to .50 when averaged over all of the subjects. As can be seen in Figures 9.1 and 9.2, this effect is primarily due to the "linear" subjects. The interaction between the type of learning the subject received and changes in dependency on the valid cue and the invalid cue is discussed next, but these results show an overall effect of adaptation to the conflict task. Subjects do adapt to the change in task structure encountered during the interactive stage of the experiment since their utilization of the cues does tend to show convergence toward a judgmental policy of equal use of the two cues.

The important interaction noted above is related to the initial learning of the subjects. For half of the subjects the valid cue was linearly related to the criterion during learning and for the other subjects the valid cue was curvilinearly related to the criterion (see the discussion in Chapter 3), and this suggests a distinct difference in the nature of the task confronting the two groups of subjects. The overall effect for the comparison of linear and nonlinear subjects is not statistically significant for either the valid-cue or invalid-cue correlations, so that for all conflict trials the use of the valid and invalid cues by subjects does not depend on whether subjects learned to use a linear or nonlinear function form.

However, there is a difference related to learning if the conflict trials are divided into blocks, and this interaction is statistically significant. The changes in dependency on the valid and invalid cues depend on whether subjects learned a linear or nonlinear function form. The interaction is significant at the .01 level for the valid cue ($F = 8.79; df = 1, 60; p < .01$) and at the .05 level for the invalid cue ($F = 4.83; df = 1, 60; p < .05$). As can be seen in Figures 9.1 and 9.2, subjects who originally learned to use a linear cue-criterion function form show a tendency to decrease dependency on that cue and to increase dependency on the other cue. This trend is not apparent for subjects who originally learned to use a curvilinear cue-criterion function form. There is also an apparent effect due to the drugs, and this effect is considered next.

## Drug Effects

There are no statistically significant main effects for the drug groups and only one significant interaction. However, there are several effects that approach statistical significance. For example, an apparent difference between drug groups for nonlinear subjects can be seen in Figure 9.2, suggesting a complex conflict (Block × Type of Learning × Drug Group) interaction. This interaction approaches statistical significance ($F = 3.09; df = 1, 40; p < .10$). The average correlation between the invalid cue and a subject's judgments increases during conflict for nonlinear subjects given methylphenidate, but decreases for subjects given pentobarbital.

These results suggest, but do not prove, an important differential effect of the two drugs that depends upon task characteristics. The group of subjects given pentobarbital, who learned to use a curvilinear function form, do *not* adapt to task characteristics during conflict since these subjects do not learn to use the invalid cue during conflict. There is a corresponding finding for the valid cue; nonlinear subjects given pentobarbital tend to maintain a higher correlation between the valid cue and their judgments than do either methylphenidate or placebo subjects, although this Subject × Drug Group interaction does not approach statistical significance ($F = 1.04; df = 2, 60; p < .25$). The trend is, however, in the direction hypothesized and is therefore further evidence for poor task adaptation by nonlinear subjects who are given pentobarbital.

The differences between the publically stated judgments of two subjects over a series of trials provide a measure of overt conflict (see Chapter 3), a measure that should be affected if the drugs differentially influence conflict reduction. An analysis of variance for overt conflict (with 5 blocks of 4 trials each as a repeated measure variable and with sex and drug group, excluding the placebo group, "between subjects" variables) shows a drug-group effect that is not significant ($F = 2.35; df = 1, 20; .25 > p > .10$), but *is* in accord with the hypotheses about drug effects. The average absolute discrepancy between the overt judgments of subjects is 3.38 for pentobarbital and 2.67 for methylphenidate; overt conflict is therefore greater with the depressant.

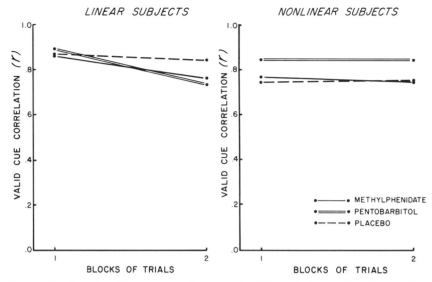

**Figure 9.1.**   Retention of dependency on the previously valid cue *r* by linear and nonlinear subjects under three drug conditions.

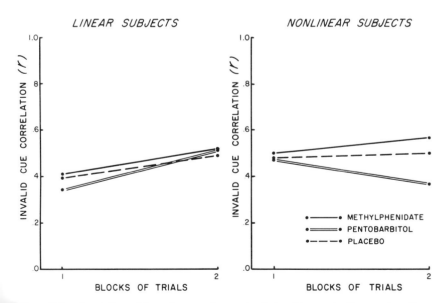

**Figure 9.2.**   Acquisition of dependency on the previously invalid cue *r* by linear and nonlinear subjects under three drug conditions.

A similar result occurs for covert conflict, the discrepancy between the private judgments of the subjects (see Chapter 3). An analysis of variance with the same factors as for overt conflict shows a nearly significant Drug Group × Sex interaction ($F = 2.73; df = 2,30; p < .10$) if all three groups, including the placebo group, are analyzed. Table 9.1 shows that this interaction is due primarily to differences between the two drug groups. The table shows quite clearly that the amount of covert conflict depends upon both the *drug* given to the subject and the *sex* of the subject, and this Drug Group × Sex interaction is statistically significant if the placebo group is excluded from the analysis ($F = 5.59; df = 1, 20; p < .05$). Table 9.1 shows that covert conflict was slightly greater for males given methylphenidate than for males given pentobarbital. For females this trend is reversed, and the difference between the two female drug groups is marked.

**Table 9.1.  Covert Conflict** [a]

|  | Methylphenidate | Pentobarbital | Placebo |
|---|---|---|---|
| Males | 1.29 | 1.13 | 1.23 |
| Females | .86 | 2.17 | 1.20 |
| Average | 1.08 | 1.65 | 1.21 |

[a]Figures represent the average absolute differences between the covert judgments of subjects for all conflict trials.

The finding that suggests the importance of the sex of the subject in moderating the effect of the drugs is not statistically reliable, but it is partially supported by interpersonal learning data (described in Chapter 12) and has important implications for the use of these drugs.

## DISCUSSION

The findings from the present study suggest that the two variables of potential importance in determining the effects of psychoactive drugs on interpersonal judgment and conflict in normal subjects are task structure and sex of the subjects. The findings with respect to drug effects are not definitive, but they are in accord with Gillis' hypothesis about the effects of stimulant and depressant drugs.

The importance of task structure is indicated by the fact that changes in the use of the valid cue and the invalid cue (cues having high and low validity during learning, respectively) during conflict depend upon whether a subject learned to use a linear or a curvilinear function form between cue and criterion. Subjects who originally learned to use a nonlinear function form were not as adaptable to task requirements during conflict as were subjects who learned to use a linear function form. This finding is important with respect to the method for studying social judgment. However, the nonsignificant trends involving drug groups are of greater importance here. As noted above, Figure 9.2 suggests that change *does* occur for nonlinear subjects during conflict trials, but that change depends upon the drug given to the subjects. Gillis' hypothesis was that subjects given a stimulant would show greater task orientation and learn more about the task than subjects given a depressant. This indeed is the case, since subjects given methylphenidate change in the direction of increasing their use of the invalid cue while use of the invalid cue declines for subjects given pentobarbital. But this is true for only the nonlinear subjects.

The result for the invalid cue is nearly statistically significant, but the nonsignificant effect that can be seen in Figure 9.1 for the valid cue is also in the hypothesized direction. Subjects who learned to use a highly valid cue in a nonlinear way continue to depend on that cue to a greater extent during conflict if they were among subjects given pentobarbital; this drug does result in lessened task adaptation.

The statistically nonsignificant drug effects for overt and covert conflict are also in the predicted direction. Since subjects given the stimulant drug were expected to be better able to learn about the task, both overt and covert judgments would be expected to converge. Measures of overt and covert conflict did show less conflict for subjects given methylphenidate when compared to subjects given pentobarbital (the marginal statistical significance of the results and the lack of firm prior hypotheses make it impossible to draw conclusions about placebo effects).

The other highly suggestive result was the indication of the importance of the sex of subjects in relation to drug effects. Covert conflict was notably higher for females given pentobarbital than for females given methylphenidate, whereas covert conflict was slightly lower for males given pentobarbital than for males given methylphenidate. The interaction between sex and drug group is an important finding. Since a similar interaction occurs for measures of interpersonal learning, it is discussed after those results are presented in Chapter 12.

In conclusion, although the results of this study are more suggestive than definitive, Gillis' hypotheses receive at least some support; additionally, task structure and sex of the subject are seen to be potentially important factors moderating the effects of the drugs. These findings provide several avenues for exploration.

# REFERENCES

Davis, K. E., Evans, W. O., and Gillis, J. S. The effects of amphetamine and chlor-promazine on cognitive skills and feelings in normal adult males. In W. O. Evans and N. Kline (Eds.), *The psychopharmacology of the normal human.* Springfield, Ill.: Charles C. Thomas, 1969.

Eysenck, H. J. Personality and drug effects. In H. J. Eysenck (Ed.), *Experiments with drugs.* London: Pergamon, 1963.

Eysenck, H. J. *The biological basis of personality.* Springfield, Ill.: Charles C. Thomas, 1967.

Gillis, J. S. and Davis, K. E. The effects of psychoactive drugs on complex thinking in paranoid and nonparanoid schizophrenics: An application of the multiple-cue model to the study of disordered thinking. In L. Rappoport and D. Summers (Eds.), *Human judgment and social interaction.* New York: Holt, Rinehart & Winston, 1973.

CHAPTER 10

# Effects of Chlorpromazine and Thiothixene on Acute Schizophrenic Patients

JOHN S. GILLIS

It has long been suspected that difficulties associated with social interaction are not only prominent symptoms of schizophrenia but also are involved in its etiology as well (Cameron, 1947; Cameron & Magaret, 1951; Clausen & Kohn, 1960; Rodnick & Garmezy, 1957; Sullivan, 1953). One of the primary functions of psychoactive chemicals employed to treat the disorder, or the several disorders, labeled "schizophrenia" should therefore be to facilitate social behavior. There is a growing, although not always consistent, body of evidence that drugs, along with their many antipsychotic effects, are successful in this regard; that is, the evidence suggests that the interpersonal behavior of schizophrenic patients is facilitated by the phenothiazines, butyrophenones, and other agents commonly used in the chemotherapy of schizophrenia (Goldberg, 1970; Klein & Davis, 1969; Klerman, 1970; May, 1968).

The main evidence concerns what might be termed the phenotypical aspects of social interaction. The drugs of choice for schizophrenics diminish withdrawal and allow such patients to be more interpersonally active on both the hospital ward and in therapeutic circumstances (Goldberg, 1970; Goldberg, Klerman, & Cole, 1965; Goldberg, Mattsson, Cole, & Klerman, 1967; Hindley, Kerin & Thompson, 1965). There is little information, however, to suggest how the drugs affect the *use* the patient makes of social interactions. Certainly there can be no benefits at all from social interactions if the patient fails to participate in them. And the use of certain drugs accomplishes an important first step simply by increasing the propensity to interact with others. Social contact per se is only a preliminary stage, however; an equally critical problem is the effect of therapeutic drugs on what patients learn from increased interpersonal contacts. It is possible to imagine, for example, a drug (alcohol comes immediately to mind) that might increase an individual's willingness to engage in social interactions, and yet markedly diminish his ability to learn anything from them. The point is critical since, regardless of how one thinks of the various psychological and milieu therapies, they obviously involve some kind of learning within an interpersonal context. Furthermore, impressive data suggests that chlorpromazine, one of the drugs most frequently used with schizophrenics, impairs learning in virtually every situation studied (Hartlage, 1965).

The purpose of this investigation was to evaluate the effects of selected antipsychotic psychoactive agents on interpersonal learning, that is to assess the role of two drugs commonly used in the treatment of schizophrenics on their ability to learn *about* other persons.

The kinds of learning in which we were interested involved subject's ability to learn about another's "cognitive system": the way in which the other person utilized information to arrive at a decision, his capacity to resolve differences with another, and his propensity to maintain a consistent approach to problems. The research paradigm employed was that described within the triple-system case in Chapter 3.

Although social learning was of primary concern data was also obtained regarding drug effects on the learning of objective tasks, specifically the judgmental learning tasks developed by Gillis (Davis, Evans, & Gillis, 1969; Gillis, 1969; Gillis, 1971; Gillis & Davis, 1973). These provided a frame of reference for the interpersonal learning data. It is possible, for example, that certain therapeutic drugs impair task learning but facilitate learning in social circumstances (this is, in fact, what might be expected from a survey of the empirical data on chlorpromazine). The objective tasks were also included because they represented in themselves promising techniques for evaluating some less apparent cognitive effects of psychoactive drugs (Gillis & Davis, 1973; see also Chapter 5 and 6).

The drugs selected for evalutaion were chlorpromazine (Thorazine) and thiothixene (Navane). The former was chosen as a representative phenothiazine because of (1) its widespread use with schizophrenics, (2) the substantial body of evidence already available regarding its clinical efficacy (Klein & Davis, 1969), (3) its consequences for learning (Hartlage, 1965), and (4) its demonstrated effects on performance with materials similar to those used in this study (Davis, Evans, & Gillis, 1969; Gillis & Davis, 1973). Thiothixene, a thioxanthene derivative, was selected as a major nonphenothiazine antipsychotic agent that has been demonstrated to be effective in the reduction of schizophrenic symptoms and that appears to be especially effective upon symptoms involving social withdrawal.

# METHOD

Details regarding (1) the design and general procedures for the study, (2) the drugs evaluated and the assignment of subjects to drug groups, and (3) characteristics of the subject sample are reported in Chapter 4. It is sufficient to repeat here that subjects were 19 adolescent schizophrenics resident on an acute treatment ward. The treatments were chlorpromazine (Thorazine) and thiothixene (Navane), and a placebo.

## Tasks and Procedure

Investigation of the effects of drugs on interpersonal learning (IPL) represented the third stage of the larger study described in Chapters 4 and 7. As noted in Chapters 3 and 4, the IPL trials follow the cognitive conflict phase.

In the third stage, subjects, after having worked together for financial rewards in 20 trials (as described in Chapter 7) were required to predict the other person's judgments over 10 additional trials. The task materials were the same as in the training and interactive stages. Subjects, after viewing each cue card (with its indications of teacher "intelligence" and "discipline"), made their judgments of "quality of teacher," and also attempted to predict the judgment the other person would make. No task outcome feedback was given during this phase. Subjects would enter their own judgment on the record sheet, enter their prediction of the other person's judgment, and proceed to the next trial. (See also Chapters 11, 12, and 13.)

Financial reinforcements were again used in this stage, each subject being paid $0.25 for each trial on which he was within $\pm$ 2 of predicting the other person's judgment correctly. Subjects could therefore earn as much as $2.50 in the third stage of the study.

## RESULTS AND DISCUSSION

Because this chapter represented the third and final stage of a larger study, segments of which are reported in Chapters 4 and 7 of this book, this discussion section includes an evaluation of the entire pattern of results from the study. In several instances, reference will be made to figures and the data considered in the earlier chapters.

## INTERPERSONAL LEARNING

### Predictive Accuracy

After subjects had interacted for the 20 trials in the joint decision stage of the study (Chapter 7), an attempt was made to assess the extent to which they had learned *about* their partner; that is, about how their partner utilized the information in making his judgments. This assessment was considered to be especially important since it provides an index of how much a subject is able to make use of a social interaction to learn something about another person directly relevant to his present situation (in this case something leading to financial rewards). The specific measure employed was "predictive accuracy," which was measured by correlating a subject's predictions of his partner's judgment on each trial with his partner's actual judgment.

This product-moment correlation between predicted and actual response was determined over the 10 IPL trials for each subject and then averaged (using Fisher's $z$-transformation) for the drug and placebo groups. The placebo subjects learned most about their partners, the chlorpromazine subjects least, and the thiothixene group was midway between the two. This is, of course, similar to the orders of proficiency obtained with the various interactive (conflict) and objective task indices (see Figure 10.1).

### Actual Similarity

In is also possible to determine from IPL data the extent to which subjects are in fact in agreement with one another (actual similarity), and the extent to which each individual sees his partner as being similar to himself (assumed similarity), regardless of whether this is actually the case. Predictive accuracy, for example, will be low for any subject who views his partner as using the same judgmental strategy as himself if his partner is really using a different policy.

Actual similarity is represented by the correlation between a subject's judgmental responses and those of his partner, and so is indicative of the extent to which subjects' policies are in agreement. These correlations were determined for each of the two drug groups and the placebo subjects. The correlations were then converted to standardized scores (Fisher's $z$-transformation), and means were determined for each group and then reconverted to average correlation coefficients (Figure 10.2). The thiothixene (Navane) and placebo subjects demonstrated somewhat more actual similarity than chlorpromazine (CPZ) subjects. Although

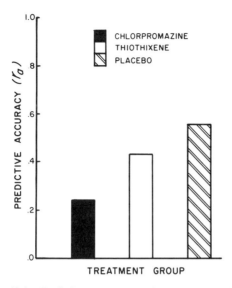

**Figure 10.1.** Predictive accuracy $r_a$ under three drug conditions.

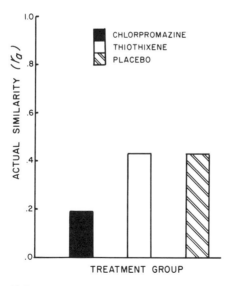

**Figure 10.2.** Actual similarity $r_a$ under three drug conditions.

this may have accounted in part for the lowered predictive accuracy of CPZ patients, the differences between the groups are not statistically significant.

## Assumed Similarity

This index, discussed in Chapter 3, represents the extent to which a subject considers the judgmental policy of his partner to be similar to his own—whether or not this is actually the case. It is determined by correlating a subject's own task judgments with his *predictions* of his partner's judgments. Mean correlations (calculated by transformations to standardized scores) were determined for the drug and placebo groups (Figure 10.3). All three groups resembled each other on this index. The antipsychotic drugs studied did not appear to affect the subjects' propensities to ascribe their own judgmental strategies to others. This tendency was pronounced for all three schizophrenic groups.

## Consistency

In the analyses of antipsychotic drug effects on objective task learning (Chapter 4) and conflict resolution (Chapter 7), much of the impairment apparently due to drug

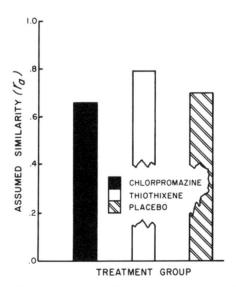

**Figure 10.3.**    Assumed similarity $r_a$ under three drug conditions.

treatment may have occurred because the subjects receiving them became less consistent in their judgmental policies. Consistency is also a critical factor in interpersonal learning. Individuals with highly inconsistent policies are difficult to learn *about*; they present unstable behavior to predict. Similarly, if one's own strategy for assessing a partner's response is itself inconsistent, one cannot achieve a high degree of accuracy.

To evaluate the effect of the drugs on consistency in the IPL trials, indices of policy stability were determined in two ways. First, the stability of a subject's own policy—that is, the consistency of his response system—was determined, and means were calculated for all treatment groups. The index of stability (described in Chapter 3) was the squared multiple correlation $R_s^2$ between a subject's responses and the actual cue values over the 10 IPL trials (Figure 10.4).

Next, the consistency of each subject in predicting his partner's response was determined by calculating the squared multiple correlation $R_p^{2\prime}$ between the cue values and his predictions of his partner's responses. Mean correlations were determined for all treatment groups (Figure 10.5). The CPZ patients evidenced least consistency in both regards—in their own judgmental systems and in their predictions of their partner's responses. The placebo group was most consistent, although this was true only when comparison was made with thiothixene (Navane) subjects in regard to the stability of their prediction strategies.

These patterns of policy stability (or "cognitive control") are indeed congruent

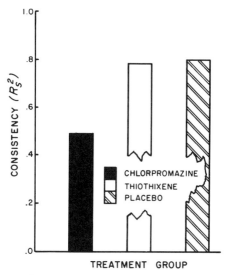

**Figure 10.4.**    Consistency $R_s^2$ of subject's own task judgment system under three drug conditions.

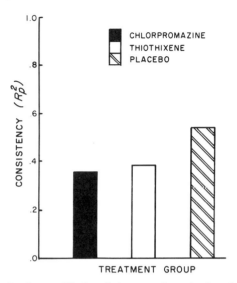

**Figure 10.5.**   Consistency  $R_p^2$  of predictive strategies under three drug conditions.

with drug group differences in predictive accuracy—and with consistency data in the task learning and conflict resolution segments of the larger investigation. They serve to re-emphasize the critical role of cognitive control in judgmental performance, and the apparent adverse effects antipsychotic drugs—or at least chlorpromazine—have on such control.

## DISCUSSION

The overall pattern of results as reported in Chapters 4 and 7, as well as with the IPL measures, is thus strikingly consistent across a variety of independent indices. Placebo subjects perform best, and are the most consistent, regardless of whether they are learning objective tasks, learning from another individual, or about another individual. Both of the drugs studied impair the performance of patients on these measures, although chlorpromazine appears to have more severe disruptive effects. The tasks used here extend previous work with schizophrenics; they are among the most complex yet evaluated with the drug. Chlorpromazine, and perhaps to a slightly lesser extent thiothixene, may generate a kind of "cognitive dampening," a diminution in the recipient's ability to bring cognitive functions effectively to bear on any complex learning situation, whether it is social or impersonal.

Finding that the impairment induced by these commonly used drugs extends to social interaction and interpersonal learning situations is important. On any view of psychotherapy various kinds of interpersonal learning must be involved. One member (the patient) is expected to learn something *from* the other (the therapist) about how to conceptualize, react to, or cope more effectively with his environment. Successful psychotherapy seems to include a good deal of learning *about* another individual as well (his values, attitudes, views of self, and the like). Such interpersonal learning appears to be impaired by the drugs studied here. The implication is straightforward—some, at least, of the psychoactive chemicals appropriately used to control psychotic *behaviors* in the schizophrenic (and there is no denying that they accomplish this important function) may nevertheless render him less susceptible to other forms of treatment, the psychological therapies involving learning more *about* and *from* other persons.

In considering how the drugs in question impaired resolution of cognitive differences and objective task learning, it was pointed out that their effect upon consistency was critical. It may be that the influence of the drugs on the consistency or "control" functions are among their most significant cognitive effects. Hammond (Chapter 3) suggests that defects in control can diminish cognitive effectiveness in a wide range of situations. Schizophrenics are generally more variable in their performance than are normals, and impaired cognitive control may simply be another manifestation of this variability in response. It would be expected that antipsychotic drugs would decrease this variability, making the patient's behavior more predictable, and would enable him to bring some subjective order into his world. However, variability in the cognitive sphere may actually be increased by the drugs in question.

Such diminished "control" could have serious implications for both interpersonal and impersonal learning. If so the consequences for the chemotherapy of schizophrenics are considerable. Effects upon learning and cognitive control, as well as individual symptoms, should be considered when choosing the treatment. In some instances, the "costs" of impairing learning abilities will have to be weighed against the alleviation of symptoms. Perhaps a specific antipsychotic drug, or combination of such drugs will be identified (or developed) that will continue to reduce symptoms without impairing cognitive functioning. Such a chemical agent is greatly needed, and perhaps may be identified more quickly by using research methods such as those described here.

## REFERENCES

Cameron, N. A. *The psychology of behavior disorders.* New York: Houghton Mifflin, 1947.

Cameron, N. A. and Magaret, A. *Behavior pathology.* New York: Houghton Mifflin, 1951.

Clausen, J. A. and Kohn, M. Social relations and schizophrenia: A research report and perspective. In D. Jackson (Ed.), *The etiology of schizophrenia.* New York: Basic Books, 1960.

Davis, K. E., Evans, W. O., and Gillis, J. S. The effects of amphetamine and chlorpromazine on cognitive skills and feelings in normal adult males. In W. O. Evans and N. Kline (Eds.), *The psychopharmacology of the normal human.* Springfield, Ill.: Charles C. Thomas, 1969.

Gillis, J. S. Schizophrenic thinking in a probabilistic situation. *Psychological Record,* 1969, **19,** 211–224.

Gillis, J. S. Ecological relevance and the study of diversed thinking. In J. Hellmuth (Ed.), *Cognitive studies,* Vol. 2. *Deficits in cognition.* New York: Brunner-Mazel, 1971.

Gillis, J. S. and Davis, K. E. The effects of psychoactive drugs on complex thinking in paranoid and nonparanoid schizophrenics: An application of the multiple-cue model to the study of disordered thinking. In L. Rappoport and D. Summers (Eds.), *Human judgment and social interaction.* New York: Holt, Rinehart & Winston, 1973.

Goldberg, S. C. Brief resume of the National Institute of Mental Health study in acute schizophrenia. In W. Clark and J. del Giudice (Eds.), *Principles of psychopharmacology.* New York: Academic, 1970.

Goldberg, S. C., Klerman, G. L., and Cole, J. O. Changes in schizophrenic psychopathology and ward behavior as a function of phenothiazine treatment. *British Journal of Psychiatry,* 1965, **111,** 120–133.

Goldberg, S. C., Mattsson, N., Cole, J. O., and Klerman, G. Prediction of improvement in schizophrenia under four phenothiazines. *Archives of General Psychiatry,* 1967, **16,** 107–117.

Hartlage, L. C. Effects of chlorpromazine on learning. *Psychological Bulletin,* 1965, **64,** 235–245.

Hindley, J. P., Kerin, M. T., and Thompson, M. Comparison of three phenothiazines on chronic psychotic behavior. *Diseases of the Nervous System,* 1965, **26,** 91–98.

Klein, D. F. and Davis, J. M. *Diagnosis and drug treatment of psychiatric disorders.* Baltimore: Williams and Wilkins, 1969.

Klerman, G. L. Clincial efficacy and actions of antipsychotics. In A. DiMascio and R. Shader (Eds.), *Clinical handbook of psychopharmacology.* New York: Science House, 1970.

May, P. R. A. *Treatment of schizophrenia.* New York: Science House, 1968.

Rodnick, E. H. and Garmezy, N. An experimental approach to the study of motivation in schizophrenia. In M. R. Jones (Ed.), *Nebraska symposium on motivation.* Lincoln University of Nebraska Press, 1957.

Sullivan, H. S. *The interpersonal theory of psychiatry.* New York: Norton, 1953.

CHAPTER 11

# Effects of Methylphenidate on Mildly Depressed Hospitalized Adults

ELLEN R. GRITZ

This study investigates the effects of methylphenidate on the same population of mildly depressed males studied in Chapters 5 and 8. The question of interest is whether methylphenidate enhances or impairs the ability of these patients to learn about another person.

Consistent with the hypotheses of facilitation of individual acquisition of the judgment task and joint learning (conflict) performance, it was proposed that methylphenidate would enhance the ability of the subjects to learn about one another. Enhanced attention and concentration or enhanced intellectual functioning would be mechanisms possible to be so affected by methylphenidate. Studies in the literature bearing on facilitation of learning by stimulants were reviewed in the beginning of Chapter 10. The evidence presented in the learning and conflict chapters of this report (Chapters 5 and 8) suggested an impairing effect of methylphenidate on various aspects of cue utilization, however.

## METHOD

Details of subjects and experimental design are specified in Chapter 5 and in Gillis (Chapter 4). Specific to this section are the interpersonal learning (IPL) trials on which subjects made individual judgments on the teacher-rating task and then guessed at his partner's judgment. Performance was evaluated by analysis, and the specific IPL measures of predictive accuracy, actual similarity, and assumed similarity (to be explained below).

## PROCEDURE

### Drugs

As detailed previously, methylphenidate hydrochloride (10 mg, t.i.d.) or placebo were each administered to two groups of subjects (14 subjects per group) for 5 days. Learning occurred on day 4 of medication and the conflict and IPL sessions on day 5 of medication.

### Task

The IPL task consisted of 10 additional cards that were presented to the subject pair. Each subject made his own judgment, and then guessed the judgment his partner had made. There was no discussion and no feedback ("correct answer").

The interpersonal conflict situation described in Chapter 8 directly preceded the interpersonal learning trials (see also Gillis, Chapter 10).

## RESULTS

### Predictive Accuracy

Predictive accuracy is the correlation between the prediction of the other by one $S$ and the actual response of the other, and it is therefore the measure of how well each subject predicted his partner's response. No significant differences between drug and placebo groups or between linear and nonlinear subjects were found on the various indices of predictive accuracy: the overall accuracy measure $r_a$, the knowledge measure $G$, or the consistency measure $R^2$ in predicting the other.

### Assumed Similarity

Assumed similarity is the analysis of how similar subjects considered themselves to be. The correlation of the judgment of $S_1$ and his prediction of the judgment of $S_2$ yielded no differences between drug and placebo groups or between linear and nonlinear subjects on any of the measures of performance $r_a$, $G$ or $R^2$.

## Actual Similarity

Actual similarity is the correlation of the private judgment of $S_1$ with that of $S_2$. There was no difference between drug and placebo groups or between linear and nonlinear $S$'s on $r_{la}$ or $G$. On $R^2$, linear subjects were significantly more consistent than nonlinear subjects ($F = 4.5456$; $df = 1, 24$; $p < .05$); however, medication had no effect.

## DISCUSSION

In the study of interpersonal conflict, methylphenidate subjects performed with improperly directed attention by maintaining dependency on the previously valid cue instead of making a judgment on the basis of both cues equally. Their performance measures of achievement and knowledge were not inferior to placebo subjects, however; these subjects were aware of the task demands and were producing overall appropriate behavior. It is not surprising, therefore, that they evidenced no deficits in interpersonal learning in the present study. On the other hand, methylphenidate did not appear to help mildly depressed patients learn about one another.

CHAPTER 12

# Effects of Methylphenidate and Barbiturate on Normal Subjects

N. ZACHARIADIS and D. VARONOS

The theory concerning the relation between stimulant and depressant drugs described in Chapter 9 in connection with interpersonal conflict is applied to the study of interpersonal learning in this chapter. And on the basis of Gillis' general theory and associated empirical studies presented in Chapters 4 and 7, the general hypothesis applied to interpersonal learning is the following: subjects who received methylphenidate will learn less about the judgmental policies of the other member of the pair than will subjects who received pentobarbital. Additionally, it would be anticipated that because of the "openness" of subjects receiving methylphenidate, they would focus less specifically on the other person, and thus be less aware of the difference between themselves and the other person; therefore, their assumed similarity scores would be higher than the scores of those receiving pentobarbital. In short, predictive accuracy in the interpersonal learning phase of the research paradigm should be lower for pairs receiving methylphenidate than for pairs receiving pentobarbital.

## METHOD

The method and procedure, including the administration of the drugs, described in detail in Chapter 9 is not reviewed here; there is, however, a brief description of the nature of the interpersonal learning task.

The interpersonal learning phase of the study involves judgments by each subject over a series of trials, as well as predictions of his partner's judgments. The interpersonal learning task involves 10 trials in which each subject gives both his own judgments and predictions of the other subject's judgments. If actual judgments are compared, a measure of the *actual similarity* between the judgmental policies of the subjects is available. A comparison of a subject's predicted judgments for the other subject with the second subject's judgment yields measures of *predictive accuracy*. And, finally, a comparison of a single subject's own judgments and his predictions of the other subject's judgments provides information about *assumed similarity* between judgmental policies. (See Chapter 3 for a discussion of these measures; other studies of interpersonal learning in this book used similar methods.)

## RESULTS

Each of the three kinds of interpersonal learning comparisons (actual similarity, predictive accuracy, and assumed similarity) provides three measures that are of relevance here ($r_a$, $G$, and $R^2$) (see Chapter 3 for a discussion of these measures). Because the results described appear to depend upon the drugs used, rather than the placebo, most of the statistical results are given only for the two drug groups.

### Assumed Similarity

Results for assumed similarity are presented first since most of the statistically significant effects involve assumed similarity. These results may be summarized by noting that there is a significant Sex × Drug Group interaction for actual similarity $r_a$ as well as for its components $G$ and $R^2$. These interactions are significant when three groups (methylphenidate, pentobarbital, and placebo) are compared or when the two drug groups (excluding the placebo group) are compared. The effect of the drugs therefore depends upon the sex of the subjects; the results are statistically reliable.

Thus, for actual similarity (the correlation between a subject's own judgment and the predicted judgments for the other subject, $r_a$), the Sex × Drug Group interaction is significant at the .05 level ($F = 5.98$; $df = 1, 40$; $p < .05$). For $G$ ($r$ corrected for unreliability in each set of judgments) the Sex × Drug Group interaction is significant at the .01 level ($F = 9.09$; $df = 1, 40$; $p < .01$). And finally, for $R^2$, the squared multiple correlation for each set of judgments, the Sex × Drug Group interaction is again statistically significant at the .01 level ($F = 8.99$; $df = 1, 88$; $p < .01$).

These interactions occur because male performance is higher with methylphenidate than pentobarbital, whereas for females the reverse is true. Performance for placebo subjects tends to be consistent across the sex factor and at about the same level as for the drug that gives the highest result for each sex.

The other statistically significant result was an effect of drug group for $r_a$ when all groups are compared, including the placebo group ($F = 5.65$; $df = 2, 60$; $p < .01$). The results for $r_a$ are shown in Figure 12.1 (since the interaction effect is similar for all three measures only values of $r_a$ are shown). For each sex, the placebo yields results comparable to results for the drug for which assumed similarity is highest. Assumed similarity is highest for *male* subjects given *pentobarbital* and for *female* subjects given *methylphenidate*.

**Actual Similarity**

There are no significant main effects or interactions for actual similarity (the correlation between the judgments of the two subjects) although there is a nonsignificant tendency for the interaction between sex of the subject and drug given. For example, the average values of $R^2$ for male subjects are .76 for those who were given methylphenidate and .88 for those who were given pentobarbital; comparable values for females are .87 and .75 ($F = 2.44$; $df = 1, 40$; $.25 > p > .10$).

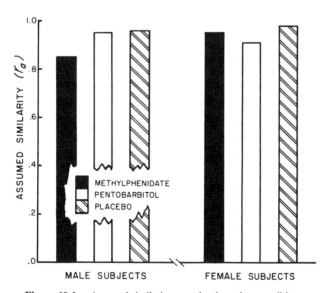

**Figure 12.1.**    Assumed similarity $r_a$ under three drug conditions.

## Predictive Accuracy

Although the Sex $\times$ Drug Group interaction is apparent for $r_a$ and $G$, it only reaches statistical significance for $R^2$, for which it is significant at the .01 level when the drug groups are compared ($F = 8.87; df = 1, 80; p < .01$). The nature of the interaction between these variables is the same as in assumed similarity.

Values of $R^2$ are computed for both predicted responses and the other subject's actual responses, and the main effect for the type of judgment is statistically significant ($F = 4.16; df = 1, 120; p < .05$) when the three groups are compared. The linear consistency of predicted responses (averaged across three groups, $R^2 = .80$) is lower than the linear consistency for actual responses ($R^2 = .86$). If only the two drug groups are compared, the effect is not statistically significant ($F = 3.34; df = 1, 80; .10 > p > .05$).

## DISCUSSION

The important finding for the interpersonal learning trials is the significant interaction between drug group and sex of the subjects that occurs for assumed similarity. Measures available for assumed similarity are (1) the correlation between the subjects' own judgments and the predicted judgments, $r_a$; (2) the correspondence between the policies, $G$; and (3) the linear predictability of the policies, $R^2$. The effect of sex on the action of the drugs for $r_a$ occurs because of differences in both $G$ and $R^2$. The interaction again occurs for $R^2$ for predictive accuracy.

It is especially important to note that the interaction found here is consistent across all of these measures, as well as consistent with the drug group interaction with sex that was found for covert conflict (Chapter 9). Females given pentobarbital, when compared to females given methylphenidate, experience more covert conflict and also make assumed similarity judgments that reflect the greater degree of conflict. The reverse is true for males, since covert conflict is less for male pair given pentobarbital than for males given methylphenidate, and male subject given pentobarbital also show higher assumed similarity than males given methylphenidate. The position of the placebo group across the various measures tends to be intermediate between the drug groups. The results do not confirm th hypothesis that pentobarbital should produce a greater predictive accuracy tha methylphenidate for all subjects.

There is, however, a study described by Eysenck (1967) which does provid evidence consonant with the present results. Munkelt (1965) administered placebo and meprobamate, a depressant drug, to male and female subjects an administered a battery of tests, including, for example, reaction time and mental arithmetic tests. She found no difference between drug and placebo groups for undifferentiated subjects, but performance for highly labile, or neurotic, subjects (as determined by use of Eysenck's Maudsley Personality Inventory; see Eysenck, 1959) was relatively lower than performance of stable subjects when the drug and placebo were compared.

Munkelt also differentiated subjects on the basis of sex, and found that female performance was lower than male performance on the test battery. Since the performance of female subjects was similar to that of the labile subjects and performance of males similar to stable subjects, a relative decrement of performance of female as opposed to male subjects would be predicted for the groups given a depressant drug. This, of course, is what occurs in the present study. The line of reasoning followed here is too tenuous to carry any further, but Eysenck's (1967) conclusion that personality and/or sex differences should be considered in assessing drug effects gains in credibility as a consequence of this comparison of Munkelt's results with those of the present study.

Finally, it should be noted that this study marks a direct attempt to discover whether interpersonal learning can be enhanced by the (acute) administration of certain psychoactive drugs. The attempt was obviously exploratory, guided primarily by Gillis' directional hypothesis about the opposing effect of stimulant and depressant drugs. The results are merely suggestive, but what they suggest is significant; interpersonal learning can be enhanced by psychoactive drugs. Additionally, however, as might be expected, the effects are apt to be influenced by biological factors (e.g., sex, detected in this study) as well as task factors (see Chapter 4 where Gillis comments on the distinction between narrow vs. wide tasks), and, of course, dose and type of drug (only two of which were used in this study).

The importance of these suggestions are two: first, the studies of drugs administered to hospitalized patients, reported in this volume, show that these drugs generally severely *impair* interpersonal learning. Therefore, it is significant that some enhancement in normals was detected, as well as no large impairment of interpersonal learning. Second, the performance of the normal subjects in the present study was quite high; the task was not difficult (only two cues were involved), and the subjects performed at about the same level as other normal subjects in the United States and Sweden in similar tasks. Therefore, any *enhancement* would be somewhat remarkable, because of the low ceiling of the task. Future research should take these findings into account by increasing the difficulty of the IPL task, thus creating a task situation more sensitive to drug effects. Of course, a wider range of drugs and doses should be investigated if possible. The need for enhanced IPL for persons whose social judgment is less than adequate is clear; whether there is a need for *drug*-enhanced IPL for normal subjects is a matter entailing ethical and moral questions as well as pragmatic ones.

## REFERENCES

Eysenck, H. J. *Manual of the Maudsley Personality Inventory*. London: University of London Press, 1959.

Eysenck, H. J. Personality and drug effects. In H. J. Eysenck (Ed.), *Experiments with drugs*. London: Pergamon, 1963.

Eysenck, H. J. *The biological basis of personality*. Springfield, Illinois: Charles C. Thomas, 1967.

Gillis, J. S. and Davis, K. E. The effects of psychoactive drugs on complex thinking in paranoid and nonparanoid schizophrenics: An application of the multiple-cue model to the study of disordered thinking. In L. Rappoport and D. Summers (Eds.), *Human judgment and social interaction*. New York: Holt, Rinehart & Winston, 1973.

Munkelt, P. Personlichkeitsmerkmale als Bedingungsfaktoren der psychotropen Argneimittelwirkung. *Psychol. Beiträge*, 1965, **8**, 98–183. Discussed in H. J. Eysenck, *The biological basis of personality*. Springfield, Illinois: Charles C. Thomas, 1967.

CHAPTER 13

# Effects of Therapeutic Dose Levels of Psychoactive Drugs on Chronic Schizophrenic Patients

JOHN S. GILLIS and CARL D. MOSS

Previous research on the effects of psychoactive drugs on social behavior has been concerned with social interaction per se. That is, a given drug has been studied with regard to the changes it produces in social interaction, such as participation in ward activities and the like. It is also possible, however, to study the use the patient makes of social interaction, to study the effects of psychoactive drugs on what may be *learned* by subjects from such interpersonal encounters (see chapters on interpersonal conflict and interpersonal learning).

Although the initial results reported above are encouraging, and the implications for drug treatment of the psychoses important, they represent only first steps. The major difficulty of the studies to date is that they lack representativeness in both task situations and drug administration. This is particularly true of the manner in which drugs are administered. The design traditionally used in psychopharmacological research has required that all subjects in a given treatment group be given *identical* dosage levels of a single drug. This group is then compared with others treated with either the same single drug at a different dosage level, or with a different single drug, or with palcebo. Thus we have acquired information about the effects of chlorpromazine, studied as a single agent, on psychotic symptoms Klein & Davis, 1969; Klerman, 1970) and on various forms of learning (Hartage, 1965).

Although this procedure adheres closely to the spirit of laboratory research, here is a price to be paid for such adherence. Such single-drug treatment groups do ot reflect current practices in psychiatric hospitals. Psychoactive drugs, including hlorpromazine, are most frequently given in *combinations*, and the dosage level

195

is *varied* according to the individual patient's needs. Comparability among patients (standardization) is effected by virtue of uniform and maximal effects on symptom diminution rather than by administering identical doses. The important questions to be asked about the cognitive consequences of the therapeutic use of antipsychotic drugs should, therefore, be directed at the effects of the dosage and combinations most frequently employed, rather than at fixed dose levels across a variety of patients. The dosage administered in empirical studies of drug effects should *not* be identical across subjects, rather, it should be the *clinically efficacious* dose for each patient. The cognitive consequences about which more should be known are those that result from drug regimes that are, in fact, chosen because they are determined to be clinically therapeutic. The price that has been paid for the use of arbitrary nonrepresentative drug study procedures is that little has been learned about the cognitive consequences of those regimes most frequently employed in the chemotherapy of schizophrenia. The present investigation, therefore, attempted to achieve greater representativeness of drug parameters by using those combinations and dosages judged by the patients' physicians to be most useful for the patients involved.

An effort was also made to move toward a more representative research situation. The conflict-interpersonal learning research paradigm used in the investigations reported in this book involves three stages: (1) learning, where two subjects learn to use information in contrasting ways; (2) subsequent conflict or interaction, where these subjects are brought together to work jointly on problems apparently similar to those they learned in the first stage; and (3) interpersonal learning, where each subject, after having worked with another individual during the interactive trials, was required to predict the responses of his partner on a further series of judgment trials (see Chapter 3). The training (learning) stage, therefore, is essential to the establishment of the cognitive differences that are the basis of the interaction between subjects. It is the learning stage that induces differences that in fact might otherwise not exist between the subjects and therefore that may introduce artificial disagreement between them. And although it is true that some investigators (Rappoport, 1969; Summers, 1968; Helenius, 1973; Brown & Hammond, 1968) have shown that essentially the same results are produced irrespective of whether subjects are trained in the laboratory to have different policies or whether such policy differences are socially induced, a question remains about the learning (training) stage when the procedure is used with *patients*.

The results of the studies referred to above were based on college student populations, and college students may very well be far more flexible about learning new ways of using information than are patients. Additionally, ther appears to be some value in studying the conflict arising from opposing views that patients bring to the task as a result of their own experience. Achieving greater representativeness of the judgments patients are apt to make not only carries intrinsic value, but also appears to be of practical value. For studying pairs of patients who bring pre-existing policy differences to the research room eliminates the need for training patients to develop different policies. And although the training (learning) data may be of value in itself (as it has been in the present studies, see Chapters 4, 5, and 6), the information it provides may not always be required. There is, then, economy of time and effort as well as greater representativeness in studying patients whose judgments differ as a result of their prior social experience, rather than as a result of training.

The present study, therefore, attempted to achieve greater representativeness with regard to *(a)* drug parameters and *(b)* the task situation by using those drug combinations and dosages that the patient's physicians had judged to be clinically most useful for the patients involved, and by pairing subjects on the basis of socially induced rather than laboratory-induced policies.

## METHOD

The investigation consisted of two major stages: (1) a policy capturing stage during which it was determined which cues a subject used in making judgments; and (2) an interpersonal learning phase where subjects having policies of varying levels of stability and opposition were brought together to attempt to learn about and to predict each other's responses. Subjects were placed in one of four groups depending on the amount of discrepancy in their policies. Pairs of subjects in these four policy groups attempted to learn to predict the responses of their partners over a series of trials. Accuracy and consistency of these predictions were compared across drug groups as well as the four policy-difference conditions. Relations between interpersonal learning measures and other cognitive parameters were also investigated.

## PROCEDURE

### Subjects

Subjects were 40 chronic schizophrenics being treated at Big Spring State Hospital, Texas. The group was representative of the generally large population of schizophrenics receiving care at this hospital and consisted of inpatients (23) as well as outpatients (17); there were 26 males and 14 females. The age range of subjects (25–57 years) was wide but again representative of the population in the hospital. The mean age was 34.8 years.

IQ test results were not available for all subjects, but information about educational level was available. Educational attainment ranged from sixth grade through two years of college with 80% of the subjects falling between 8 and 11 years of formal education.

Past research (Gillis, 1969; Gillis & Davis, 1973) has suggested that variables such as age, education, and intelligence do not affect performance on the kinds of tasks used in this study. Therefore no attempt was made to control for these variables across drug and task conditions; assignment to the latter was based on a subject's judgmental policy, his particular drug regime having been determined by his physician. Nevertheless, there were no statistically significant differences between task or drug groups with regard to either age or education.

The judgment policies of 116 patients were ascertained with regard to the judgment task.

### Interactive (Policy Difference) Conditions

Four interactive conditions were established for pairs of subjects attempting to predict each other's judgmental responses. As can be seen from Table 13.1, the greatest difference between $Ss$ was represented in Condition I, the *strong differences* group. Members of the seven pairs in this condition were highly consistent ($R^2 > .80$, the measure of policy stability) and had highly contrasting policies; that is, one member depended heavily on Cue 1 (intelligence) but ignored Cue 2 (interest in patient), and the other member of the pair used only Cue 2, but gave essentially no weight to Cue 1.

Condition II was designated a *moderate difference* group. It is similar to Condition I in that the members of each pair are clearly dependent on opposing cues, but differs from I in that policies are less consistent ($R^2$ ranged from .5 through .79).

Condition III was composed of pairs of subjects who gave approximately *equal weight* to each of the two cues. Policies in this condition were highly stable, $R^2$ being above .75 for each subject.

Condition IV is referred to as the *"no policy"* group since it consisted of subjects not having consistent ways of dealing with the task ($R^2 < .42$), and thus weighting *neither* of the cues heavily.

**Table 13.1.   Distribution of Subjects by Drug Conditions and Policy Difference Groups**

| | Policy Condition | | | | |
|---|---|---|---|---|---|
| Drug Group | I<br>Strong<br>Differences | II<br>Moderate<br>Differences | III<br>Equal<br>Weights | IV<br>No<br>Policy | Total<br>$n$ |
| Thioridazine | 4 | 4 | 3 | 2 | 13 |
| Trifluoperazine | 3 | 4 | 1 | 0 | 8 |
| Haloperidol | 3 | 3 | 2 | 4 | 12 |
| Combinations | 3 | 3 | 0 | 1 | 7 |
| Total | 13 | 14 | 6 | 7 | 40 |

## Tasks

As noted above, the study involved two major phases, a policy capturing stage and an interactive stage. Since an individual's judgment policy with regard to an important issue had to be determined, task content became a critical consideration. It was necessary that a task be selected about which our sample, chronic schizophrenics in this case, would be likely to have a judgment policy. And although the "teacher task" had served well in our earlier drug-interpersonal learning work (Gillis, Chapters 4, 7, and 10), the teacher-quality criterion appeared to be too remote a concept for this study. It seemed doubtful that many chronic schizophrenics would in fact have a consistent policy regarding variables critical to the quality of teachers. On the other hand, *doctors* obviously play a vital role in the everyday life and ultimate fate of patients, and, therefore, it seemed quite likely that patients would be prepared to make judgments regarding the qualities that produce an effective doctor.

After considerable pilot work a two-cue task was developed, involving 30 trials, and which required subjects to evaluate the "quality" of various doctors. Such judgments could be made on the basis of two items of information pertaining to each doctor: *(a)* his intelligence and *(b)* his degree of interest in patients. Pilot data indicated that, using such a task, it was possible to identify subjects within a population of chronic schizophrenics, having both *consistent* and *contrasting* policies.

No task outcome feedback was given in this study; subjects could not be "incorrect" regardless of how they used the cues.

## Details of Tasks and Procedure

The tasks required subjects to make judgments of the "quality of a doctor" on the basis of two cues—"intelligence" and "interest in patients." Each of these cues had possible values ranging from 1 to 10, while criterion values (the doctor's quality) ranged from 1 to 20. The actual cue values on each trial were indicated by the height of two vertical scales or columns. During the interactive interpersonal learning (IPL) phase, subjects completed 40 trials, making two judgments on each trial: (1) their own assessment of the quality of the doctor and (2) their prediction of the judgment that their partners would make. After first recording their own judgment, subjects were free to discuss both their responses and the reasons for them. It was through such interactions, of course, that interpersonal learning could take place.

Because of the ever present problem of motivation in research with chronic schizophrenics, subjects were given financial incentives for IPL performance. Subjects were paid $0.20 for each of the last 20 interactive trials in which their prediction of the partner's response was within ± 2 points of his partner's actual answer. It was thus possible for a subject to earn up to $4.00 on Block 2 of the experiment. All subjects were paid, in addition, $1.00 for participating in the study. Such financial incentives greatly enhance the performance of acute schizophrenics on a variety of judgment tasks (see Chapter 7).

## Psychiatric Ratings

In addition to determining the consequences of antipsychotic drugs on interpersonal learning (IPL), we were also concerned with the relation between IPL and the more traditional measures of drug effectiveness. Each subject had a psychiatric interview and evaluation immediately following his IPL testing. Ratings were completed on the Inpatient Multidimensional Psychiatric Scale, IMPS (Lorr, Klett, McNair, & Lasky, 1962), after the subject had been interviewed by an experienced clinical psychologist. The ratings were made in ignorance of the medication a given subject was receiving and the subject's performance on the IPL task.

Interviews ranged from 30 minutes to 1 hour, as necessary to complete the rating form. The IMPS, which includes items relating to cognitive, emotional, and behavioral symptoms, frequently has been used to evaluate phenothiazine and other antipsychotic drug effects with schizophrenics (Goldberg, Klerman, & Cole, 1965; Goldberg, Mattsson, Cole, & Klerman, 1967).

# Drugs

The drugs they were receiving did not determine whether patients were included in the study. Each subject remained on those antipsychotic drugs and dosage levels which the physician had determined to be clinically efficacious for him. Once the performance on the IPL measures had been assessed for a considerable number of subjects, an attempt was made to compare the performances of groups of patients on similar drug regimens.

Many patients were found to be receiving more than one antipsychotic agent. In most cases, one of these agents was considered to be the *major* drug used—that is, one drug was given at a dose relatively higher than that of any other drugs the patient was receiving. Such patients were considered to belong to the drug group labeled with their major antipsychotic agent. Thus the thioridazine (Mellaril) group included 13 patients whose major drug treatment was thioridazine although some patients ($n = 5$) were receiving additional antipsychotic medication in relatively smaller doses.

Three groups of patients, each receiving different major antipsychotic drugs, were set up in this way. Several other patients were receiving antipsychotic drugs at approximately equally effective dosage levels. These patients consituted a fourth group representing "combinations" of antipsychotic agents.

There were, then, four drug groups: (1) thioridazine (Mellaril), $n = 13$; (2) trifluoperazine (Stelazine), $n = 8$; (3) haloperidol (Haldol), $n = 12$; and (4) a "combinations" group, $n = 7$. The regimes finally compared can be thought of as a reasonably representative sample of those used with psychotic patients at the facility, according to post experimental discussion with the hospital staff.

# RESULTS

Because of the manner in which subjects were selected for the study (nature and stability of policy) it was not possible to accomplish a complete factorial design (4 Drug Conditions × 4 Policy Groups × 2 Learning Blocks) as originally planned. Certain of the cells in this design (especially in Policy Conditions III and IV) contained fewer than two subjects, and no cells in Policy Condition III included more than three subjects (see Table 13.1). Two alternative types of analysis were possible, however: the first compared only the first two policy groups (i.e., the "strong" and "moderate" differences groups) across all four drug conditions; the second compared all four policy groups across only two drug conditions (thioridazine and haloperidol). While the former was considered to be the more important since the cell sizes were larger (Table 13.1), both types of analysis were utilized for each comparison described below.

## INTERPERSONAL LEARNING MEASURES

### Predictive Accuracy

Over a series of 40 trials (analyzed as 2 blocks of 20 trials each) each member of the pair was required (1) to make a judgment as to quality of the "doctor" represented on the card, and (2) to predict the responses of the other person. The predictive accuracy of a subject was assessed by correlating his predictions of his partner's response with the partner's actual responses over a series of trials.

### *Achievement*

The product-moment correlations were determined over the two blocks of trials, converted to standardized scores (Fisher's $z$-transformations), and then averaged for each of the four drug groups in each of the first two policy conditions. The mean correlations are described separately for the strong and moderate policy difference groups in Figure 13.1. A $4 \times 2 \times 2$ analysis of variance (Drug Group $\times$

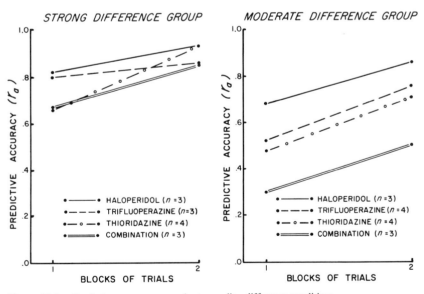

**Figure 13.1.**   Predictive accuracy $r_a$ under two policy difference conditions.

Policy Condition × Blocks of Trials) of these accuracy scores yielded significant main effects for drugs ($F = 4.75$; $df = 3$, $19$; $p < .05$), policy conditions ($F = 23.65$; $df = 1$, $19$; $p < .01$) and blocks ($F = 36.5$; $df = 1$, $19$; $p < .01$).

The block effects indicate that significant improvement occurred in predictive accuracy over trials; subjects learned to predict their partner's responses more accurately in both task conditions and in each of the four drug groups. The significant main effect for policy groups reflects the superior performance of those subjects in the strong differences condition. Although the order of performance of drug groups varies in the two task conditions, haloperidol subjects perform best in both tasks, and the "combinations" group is generally the least effective.

## Knowledge and Control

Since all three variables of interest yielded significant differences on predictive accuracy the origin of such differences was sought. Were drug differences, for example, traceable to their effects on *knowledge* about another person's judgmental system, or on the ability of the judge to implement (control) such knowledge effectively? (See Chapter 3 for details concerning these components.)

Knowledge $G$ was assessed for each subject and the scores submitted to a $4 \times 2 \times 2$ analysis of variance, similar to that performed on the achievement scores. The results demonstrated no significant main effects or interactions (Figure 13.2).

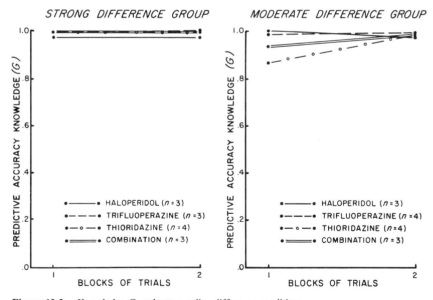

**Figure 13.2.**    Knowledge $G$ under two policy difference conditions.

Control $R^2$ scores were also determined for each subject, and an analysis of variance was accomplished over the first two policy difference conditions. Significant main effects were obtained for policy groups ($F = 6.47; df = 1, 19; p < .05$) and blocks ($F = 42.3; df = 1, 19; p < .01$) but not for drug groups (Figure 13.3).

Although significant drug group differences were not obtained on *either* component, haloperidol subjects were most effective on *both* components, as they were on overall predictive accuracy.

## Actual Similarity

As described by Hammond (Chapter 3), actual similarity is represented by the correlation between a subject's judgmental responses and those of his partner. It is therefore indicative of the extent to which members of a pair are in agreement. Actual similarity correlations were calculated across all drug groups and for the first two policy conditions (Figure 13.4). An analysis of variance of these (standardized) correlation coefficients yielded a significant main effect only for blocks of trials ($F = 24.6; df = 1, 19; p < .01$), indicating that subjects did in fact become more similar while working jointly on the tasks.

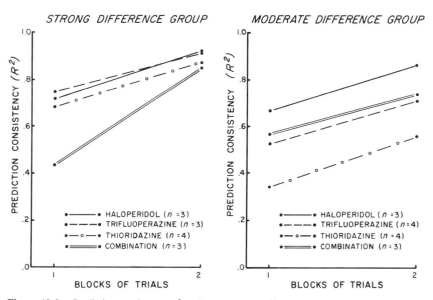

**Figure 13.3.**    Prediction consistency $R^2$ under two policy difference conditions.

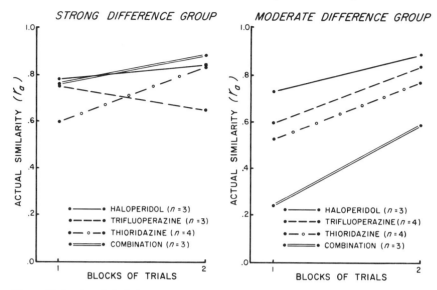

**Figure 13.4.**    Actual similarity $r_a$ under two policy difference conditions.

## Assumed Similarity

This index represents the extent to which a subject considers the judgmental policy of his partner to be similar to his own—whether or not this is actually the case. It is determined by correlating a subject's judgments with his predictions of his partner's responses. These correlations were determined for each subject and converted to $z$-scores: an analysis of variance was carried out on the resulting standardized scores. There were no significant main effects or interactions (Figure 13.5). This is important; it means that predictive accuracy was a function of *actual* similarity, not *assumed* similarity.

## Analyses under Four Conditions

The analyses of IPL performance were carried out across all four drug groups for the two policy conditions—strong and moderate differences. It was also possible to analyze data over all four policy conditions (the ''equal weight'' and ''no policy'' groups being added) if only two drugs (thioridazine and haloperidol) were compared. Such analyses were carried out for predictive accuracy, actual similarity, assumed similarity and the component indices (knowledge and control) of each.

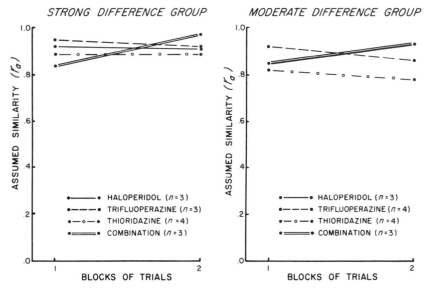

**Figure 13.5.**    Assumed similarity $r_a$ under two policy difference conditions.

### Predictive Accuracy

Significant effects were obtained with regard to predictive accuracy for blocks ($F = 41.7; df = 1, 17; p < .01$), policy conditions ($F = 8.4; df = 3, 17; p < .01$) and the Block × Policy Group interaction ($F = 3.9; df = 3, 17; p < .05$) (Figure 13.6). Similar analyses (2 Drug Groups × 4 Policy Conditions) of the knowledge and control components of accuracy did yield significant interactions involving drug groups. Thus on knowledge $G$ a significant Drug × Blocks interaction ($F = 8.5; df = 1, 17; p < .01$) reflected more rapid initial learning by haloperidol subjects (higher block 1 scores, although block 2 scores were nearly identical across policy conditions). Analysis of control scores yielded an almost significant ($F = 3.12; df = 3, 17; p > .05$) Drug × Policy Condition interaction. This was traceable to the superiority of the haloperidol subjects in the moderate differences condition (resembling the predictive accuracy results in Figure 13.6) and to the more effective performance by the thioridazine group in the "no policy" condition.

### Prior Policy Stability and Subsequent Predictive Accuracy

The analyses described thus far have examined the possibilities of predicting IPL performance from knowledge of an individual's drug group and the extent of hi~

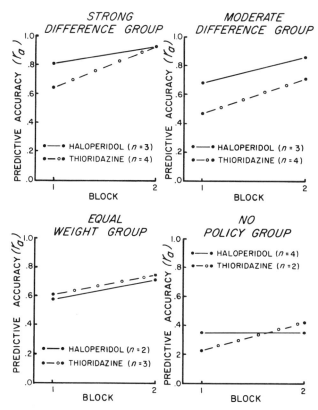

**Figure 13.6.**  Predictive accuracy $r_a$ of two drug groups under four policy difference conditions.

policy differences with a partner. Another possible set of predictors of IPL performance consists of those indices of cognitive functioning obtained *before* a subject began to work with another person. Predictive accuracy, for example, might well be correlated with prior stability during the policy capturing trials.

In order to evaluate the predictive utility of this index of cognitive behavior, the correlation between predictive accuracy scores and a subject's consistency $R^2$ during the policy capturing trials was determined. Across all subjects in the investigation, the prior $R^2$ correlated .62 with accuracy scores on block 1 and .92 with accuracy scores on block 2.

## Prior Consistency and Subsequent Consistency

The results indicated above that predictive accuracy could be predicted from an individual's policy stability $R^2$ score prior to the IPL trials. That is, one aspect of cognitive performance in an interactive situation (a two-system case) was predictable from a cognitive index obtained in an isolated judgment situation (single-system case). These relationships, although impressive, may in fact have understated the value of $R^2$ for predicting IPL performance, since predictive accuracy is dependent not only on the cognitive system of the subject of interest (the individual whose IPL performance is to be predicted) but also that of his partner. A more realistic parameter of IPL performance that might be predicted is the patient's own consistency. Consistency in IPL performance $R^2$ was therefore correlated with consistency in the policy capturing trials over all subjects. The resulting correlations were .53 with $R^2$ in block 1 and .70 with $R^2$ in block 2 of the IPL trials. Consistency during policy capturing trials—an impersonal circumstance—thus effectively predicted two major dimensions of IPL performance, consistency (control) and predictive accuracy. Very little can be said about the meaning of these results at this point, other than to observe that these relations should be studied further.

**Psychiatric Ratings**

The presence and severity of psychiatric symptoms in the sample was determined by ratings, based on interviews, on the Inpatient Multidimensional Psychiatric Scale (IMPS). The status of each drug group was assessed in two ways: (1) the ratings of all subjects in a given drug group were averaged for *each* of the 89 items on the IMPS. These average scores on individual items were then compared by multiple *t*-tests, across drug groups. (2) Items were grouped according to the fourteen symptom scales generated by factor analysis of the IMPS (Goldberg, Cole, & Clyde, 1963). Total scores on each symptom category were then compared across the four drug groups.

Neither set of analyses yielded significant drug group differences, and average scores on most IMPS items were low (53 of the 65 scaled items yielded averages under 2 on a 1–8 scale of severity). Psychiatric symptoms were thus at a very low level in our sample across all four drug regimens, as was to be expected because only patients already being successfully treated were included in the study.

**SUMMARY AND DISCUSSION**

This investigation, using representative tasks and representative antipsychotic drug regimes, allowed an evaluation of the influence of several variables on the ability of schizophrenic subjects to learn about one another. The principal pattern of the results is clear. Interpersonal learning is critically affected by: (1) the drug regimen a psychotic patient is receiving; and (2) the extent to which his policy is stable and differs from that of the individual he is attempting to assess. Further, an individual's ability to predict his partner's responses accurately can be predicted by prior knowledge of the stability of his policy when working alone on a similar judgmental task.

## Drug Effects

The differential effects of drugs on interpersonal learning are particularly striking in that they occur within a sample of patients whose symptoms were approximately equal and of minimal severity. Only those patients who were on a stable "therapeutic" dose level (including combinations of drugs) were included in the study. Each patient was on that regimen deemed, on clinical grounds, to be most successful for him in diminishing his psychotic symptoms. Data from independent psychiatric ratings supported the validity of the therapeutic value of the various drug regimes. In short, despite their *equal* influence on individual *symptoms,* the antipsychotic agents were *differentially* effective in facilitating *interpersonal learning.*

The implications of these results are considerable. They suggest that even when antipsychotic drugs do not differ in the extent to which they alleviate individual symptoms, they may nevertheless exert significantly different effects on an individual's ability to learn about another person. But as suggested above—and in other chapters in this book—interpersonal learning includes elements basic to all forms of psychological therapy. It would appear, therefore, that selection of an antipsychotic agent appropriate to the individual patient should involve its effect on IPL *in addition to* its potential for symptom alleviation. Given a variety of drugs that affect control of psychotic symptoms, differential effects on IPL might become critical in the choice of treatment.

It is noteworthy that subjects in all groups improved their ability to predict the judgments of the other person. Although it might be expected that ability to predict another person's judgmental responses would improve as a function of experience with the other person, it should be remembered that the subjects under study were hospitalized chronic schizophrenics. The improvement in the accuracy of their predictions of another psychotic subject (having in some cases a totally different approach to judgmental issues) is encouraging. Since this occurred in all drug groups, although not under all policy conditions, it appears that interpersonal learning can still occur when an individual is under treatment with any of the drug regimes studied in this experiment. Such learning is not equal across different drug groups, however, as Figure 13.1 clearly illustrates.

## Cognitive Factors

It was also to be expected that cognitive factors, such as policy differences, would be critical to IPL. Performance of all groups improves as initial differences between partners increase (Figure 13.1) and, most importantly, as policies become more predictable (Figures 13.1 and 13.6). Although the finding that *accuracy improves* as *differences increase* may appear somewhat surprising, it is to be expected, since the strong differences groups are also those having greatest policy stability. Indeed the "no policy" condition, where even the haloperidol subjects perform poorly, afforded little chance for accurate interpersonal predictions; the strategies of participants were so unstable that there was little opportunity for accuracy. The learning that does occur is due to a minimal increase in policy stability during the IPL trials—a finding that deserves further research.

Perhaps the most important aspect of the effects of cognitive factors on IPL is that differences in IPL are produced by differences in *cognitive control*. As Figure 13.2 suggests, there are essentially no differences across policy conditions on the knowledge index of performance $G$. In both conditions (and across all four drug groups), $G$ is close to 1.0. When control $R^2$ is examined (Figure 13.3), however, the reason for the differential accuracy between the "strong" and "moderate" conditions becomes clear. Where differences are strong and policies highly stable, circumstances permit considerable interpersonal learning. Where stability is diminished by even a relatively very small extent—as in the "moderate" condition—IPL suffers significantly. As Figure 13.3 indicates, these drugs facilitate IPL because they facilitate cognitive control. Although no significant main effect for drugs occurred with regard to cognitive control $R^2$, the differences among drug groups are marked and parallel the predictive accuracy results.

A further result supporting the importance of cognitive control concerns the correlations between stability during the initial "policy capturing" trials and stability as well as predictive accuracy in the IPL trials. In this case cognitive performance in an interpersonal situation (two-system case) was predicted by a cognitive measure obtained from a judgment task (one-system case). The findings suggest that an individual's capacity to learn in a social context can be predicted from knowing how he performs in a situation requiring impersonal judgment. Moreover, the particular aspect of his performance that appears to be critical for successful learning is the stability of his policy. Subjects having stable, consistent approaches to problems are those who most readily learn about others in an interpersonal situation.

The implications of this result for psychological therapies are noteworthy. To the extent that such therapies involve interpersonal learning, as we have argued they do, one might take a significant step toward predicting those patients most likely to benefit from psychotherapy by first discovering whether they are able to function in a stable, consistent manner in judgment tasks. Much the same argument can be made for prediction of probable outcome under treatment with drugs, the major focus of this investigation. Working from knowledge of the effects of various antipsychotic agents on IPL, selection of the appropriate chemical regime could be made taking into consideration both symptom alleviation *and* the extent to which the individual would be involved in psychological therapy.

While the substantive findings of this study appear to be valuable, perhaps its design is its most important aspect. An attempt was made to move toward a more representative situation for evaluating drug effects by (1) using "therapeutic" doses and combinations of drugs and (2) working with "socially induced" rather than "laboratory induced" policies. The innovations regarding assignment of drugs appear to be most important. It was decided that the most useful information regarding the effects of antipsychotic drugs on interpersonal learning could be obtained if patients were tested on those doses and combinations determined by their physicians to be clinically therapeutic. The vital question is: what happens to interpersonal learning when patients are placed on those individualized antipsychotic drug regimes that reduce their symptoms? The results, as noted, suggest that various drugs and combinations given at levels that effectively reduce symptoms, have differential consequences for interpersonal learning.

Aside from allowing an evaluation of IPL under conditions representative of actual drug treatment situations, this procedure has a further practical advantage of considerable importance. It permits easy access to an institutionalized sample, while causing minimal interference with hospital routine. Patients do not have to be put on arbitrarily selected levels of single drugs which would not otherwise be administered to them.

There are, however, liabilities associated with the strategy as well. Most important are those involving the assignment of patients to treatment groups. Rather than having all patients in a given treatment group receiving precisely the same dose of an identical drug, the "therapeutic doses" strategy results in treatment groups in which patients are receiving *different* levels of the same drug or, worse still, treatment groups in which the same drug is used in combination with a variety of other drugs. The "thioridazine plus," "trifluoperazine plus" groups in this study involved just such combinations. Standardization within groups is attained not in uniform drug regimes, but in terms of effecting minimal levels of psychiatric symptoms. It is, therefore, impossible to make cause-effect inferences with regard to specific drugs.

The assets of representativeness seem to outweigh its liabilities, because the critical question to be asked about drug effects concerns their employment in actual treatment circumstances. There is little value, for example, in knowing the consequences for learning when chlorpromazine is used alone if in fact it is rarely given without being combined with other drugs. As with much psychological research, however, moving toward more ecologically representative designs involves certain costs in precision. When evaluating the effects of psychoactive drugs the relevance of the findings seem to justify this cost.

Representativeness was also sought in making socially induced rather than laboratory-induced policies the objects of study. Although previous research had noted no essential differences between these approaches in the way they affected conflict resolution and interpersonal learning, it was decided that patients' socially induced policies might be more stable than patients' laboratory-induced policies. However, the procedural difficulties of using socially induced policies suggest the laboratory induction techniques may in fact be more practical, for several reasons. First, it is necessary to locate issues about which subjects are likely to have *stable* policies—not an easy task with hospitalized schizophrenic patients—and to find *different* policies in the sample used. Therefore, in order to select and pair subjects for the interactive phase of the experiment, large numbers of patients have to be tested in a "policy-capturing" stage. This is time consuming and costly, and perhaps only a small proportion of the subjects tested are appropriate for the interactive phase. Also, pairing subjects appropriately can be as difficult as locating persons with consistent policies.

Because (1) there was no direct comparison of socially induced and laboratory-induced policies in this study; (2) research with psychiatrically normal subjects suggests that the two types of induction do not differentially affect IPL; and (3) there are many practical problems when socially induced policies are used, it is advisable that laboratory methods of creating stable policy differences be used in future research. Whereas the attempt to be more representative with regard to drug parameters appears worth the methodological costs, this is not true with regard to the variations in task parameters attempted here.

## REFERENCES

Brown, L. and Hammond, K. R. A supra-linguistic method for reducing intragroup conflict. Unpublished manuscript, University of Colorado, Institute of Behavioral

Science, Program of Research on Human Judgment and Social Interaction, Report No. 108, 1968.

Davis, K., Evans, W. O. and Gillis, J. S. The effects of amphetamine and chlorpromazine on cognitive skills and feelings in normal adult males. In W. Evans and N. Kline (Eds.) *The psychopharmacology of the normal human.* Springfield, Ill.: Charles C. Thomas, 1969.

Gillis, J. S. Schizophrenic thinking in a probabilistic situation. *Psychological Record,* 1969, **19,** 211–224.

Gillis, J. S. and Davis, K. The effects of amphetamine and chlorpromazine on complex thinking in paranoid and nonparanoid schizophrenics. In L. Rappoport and D. Summers (Eds.), *Human judgment and social interaction.* New York: Holt, Rinehart & Winston, 1973.

Goldberg, S. C., Mattsson, N., Cole, J. O., and Klerman, G. Prediction of improvement in schizophrenia under four phenothiazines. *Archives of General Psychiatry,* 1967, **16,** 107–117.

Goldberg, S. C., Cole, J. O., and Clyde, D. J. Factor analyses of ratings of schizophrenic behavior. *Psychopharmacology Service Center Bulletin,* 1963, **2,** 23–28.

Goldberg, S. C., Klerman, G., and Cole, J. O. Changes in schizophrenic psychopathology and ward behavior as a function of phenothiazine treatment. *The British Journal of Psychiatry,* 1965, **111,** 120–133.

Hartlage, L. C. Effects of chlorpromazine on learning. *Psychological Bulletin,* 1965, **64,** 235–245.

Helenius, M. Socially induced cognitive conflict: A study of disagreement over childrearing policies. In L. Rappoport and D. Summers (Eds.), *Human judgment and social interaction.* New York: Holt, Rinehart & Winston, 1973.

Klein, D. F. and Davis, J. M. *Diagnosis and drug treatment of psychiatric disorders.* Baltimore: Williams and Wilkins, 1969.

Klerman, G. L. Clinical efficacy and actions of antipsychotics. In A. DiMascio and R. Shader (Eds.), *Clinical handbook of psychopharmacology.* New York: Science House, 1970.

Lorr, M., Klett, C. J., McNair, D. M., and Lasky, J. J. *Inpatient Multidimensional Psychiatric Scale (IMPS) Manual.* Palo Alto, Calif.: Consulting Psychologists Press, 1962.

Rappoport, L. Cognitive conflict as a function of socially-induced cognitive differences. *Journal of Conflict Resolution,* 1969, **13,** 143–148.

Summers, D. A. Conflict, compromise and belief change in a decision-making task. *Journal of Conflict Resolution,* 1968, **2,** 215–221.

# PART III

# New Directions

Of the many results discussed in Part II, it is clear that the concept of cognitive control emerges as one that carries considerable significance for the study of human judgment. Efforts to understand the cognitive dynamics of interpersonal conflict arising from differing judgments, as well as the cognitive dynamics of interpersonal learning might well take this concept into consideration. In Part III, two studies address the matter of cognitive control directly. The first reports on the use of new methods for providing cognitively oriented feedback, and the effect of such feedback on cognitive control. The second brings the concept of cognitive control under analysis in a study of the effects of methadone on judgment. A third chapter illustrates the role of cognitive control in physicians' judgments of the effects of drugs in clinical trials. Finally, some observations are made concerning future research concerning psychoactive drugs and human judgment.

CHAPTER 14

# New Procedures: Use of Interactive Computer Graphics Terminals with Psychiatric Patients

JOHN S. GILLIS, THOMAS R. STEWART, and ELLEN R. GRITZ

As progress is made in the study of human judgment the critical role of the nature and source of feedback is becoming apparent. This is particularly so with individuals attempting to improve their judgments, whether such improvement is measured by greater accuracy in the prediction of a criterion, increased similarity with the judgmental strategy of an "expert," or simply similarity with those persons not hospitalized. One technique for aiding persons to improve their judgments involves computer-mediated visual feedback. This technique provides "cognitive feedback"; it presents subjects with visual displays of both (1) their own judgmental approaches to problems, and (2) the most effective or desirable strategies, thus enabling the subjects to compare what they *should be* doing with what they *are* doing. Such methods have been demonstrated to significantly improve both the rate and degree of learning (Hammond, 1971).

The procedural details of this technique have been described elsewhere (Hammond & Summers, 1972; see also Chapter 3 of this book). It is sufficient here to summarize briefly the method and its utilities.

The advantages of the interactive computer graphics method derive mainly from its capacity to present subjects with a pictorial, easy-to-grasp description of their own approach to judgment tasks. Traditional studies of judgmental learning have depended solely upon outcome feedback to enhance performance. Subjects are informed after each trial whether or not they are correct or how closely they approached the correct answer. They are never made aware, however, of *how* their particular level of accuracy was attained—of how, for example, they effectively used or misused various items of information. The interactive computer graphics

217

technique, on the other hand, after a series of trials, provides the subjects with visual information concerning both the weights they have given various cues and the functional relationships they have employed in relating each cue to the criterion. Such *cognitive feedback* is presented in conjunction with displays of the weights and functional relationships that will lead to maximally effective performance. The characteristics of a subject's judgmental policy are thus made explicit, and related very clearly to task properties. The subject can directly observe the details of *how* he is making his judgments and how he must modify his strategy to be more accurate.

Although such an approach to feedback might be thought to enhance learning in a variety of contexts, it should be especially effective where tasks are characterized by (1) irreducible uncertainty, (2) the presence of several cues, each of which is related to the criterion in a probabilistic manner, and (3) different functional relationships between each cue and the condition to be inferred. These circumstances are representative of a variety of social judgment situations, and therefore are also properties of the kinds of tasks utilized in the present investigation of the effects of psychoactive drugs on social judgment. The benefits of interactive computer graphics methods for this work thus derive from their demonstrated capacity to facilitate learning in precisely the kinds of circumstances critical to social judgment.

Hammond (Chapter 3) has pointed out the importance of distinguishing between the knowledge and control components of performance. Effectiveness in social judgment tasks derives from (1) the extent to which a subject's policy is isomorphic with the characteristics of the environment (knowledge), and (2) the consistency with which he implements this policy (control). As noted, the major advantage of the graphics technique is that it allows a very clear display of task characteristics. Subjects can be shown in graphic form the ecologically valid cue weights and function forms. They can be shown task properties in such a way as to *maximize knowledge*. Since this is the case, interactive computer graphics methods are uniquely suited to studying the cognitive control component of performance. If, that is, precise information regarding task properties can be displayed in a form likely to maximize knowledge, performance differentials between individuals should come to depend increasingly on the consistency, or control, component. If psychoactive drugs differentially affect control, this should become most apparent when subjects learn with the assistance of interactive computer graphics methods.

The three experiments described below focused primarily on control. Task parameters—cue weights and function forms—were presented to subjects *before* they began learning trials. Knowledge was expected to be enhanced, and differ ences between drug and nondrug groups were expected to be primarily dependent on differences in control—the ability to consistently implement a known policy.

## METHOD

This exploratory work on the use of interactive computer graphics techniques for studying drug effects on learning was divided into three major studies. (1) In Experiment I, subjects from two different psychopathological populations —hospitalized schizophrenics receiving antipsychotic drugs and drug-addicted outpatients receiving methadone—and a control group of psychiatric aides dealt with four judgmental learning tasks of various levels of difficulty. Although computer-assisted visual displays were used to present stimulus materials, subjects were not given feedback except after the completion of the learning trials. Study 1, then, focused primarily on the efficacy of the graphics technique as a means of presenting stimulus materials to subjects difficult to study; subjects with whom motivation to perform has traditionally been recognized as a serious problem.

(2) Experiment II focused somewhat more on the interactive computer graphics method as a feedback device. In this study only schizophrenics and controls were used. The primary changes from Experiment I concerned task characteristics; specifically *(a)* content was added so that subjects now made judgments about a substantive issue, and *(b)* subjects received the kinds of visual feedback discussed above—feedback regarding their own judgmental policies and how these fitted task properties.

(3) Experiment III directly attacked the question of the value of cognitive feedback for schizophrenic subjects. The efficacy of three different types of task information—outcome results, task characteristics (feedforward), and cognitive feedback—was compared. While knowledge and control parameters were examined in all three studies, task information and instructions were always presented so as to maximize knowledge. Focus was thus maintained on the differential role of drugs in effecting cognitive control under the three conditions.

## Subjects

The schizophrenic sample consisted of 37 chronic inpatients at Big Spring (Texas) State Hospital. Eleven of these patients participated in Experiment I, 9 in Experiment II, and 17 in Experiment III. No effort was made to match these subjects with methadone or control groups on age, education, or IQ, although the two schizophrenic groups compared in Experiment II were matched with each other on each of these variables. (Gillis, 1969; and Gillis & Davis, 1973, found no significant relationships between any of these variables and performance on judgmental learning tasks.) In order to negate transfer effects, no subject participated in more than one study.

All schizophrenic patients were receiving antipsychotic medication; the major agents used being haloperidol (Haldol) and trifluoperazine (Stelazine). The sample was selected in such a manner that approximately half of the patients in each of the first two experiments were receiving one of these two agents as their major antipsychotic drug. Thus, of the 11 schizophrenic patients in Experiment I, 6 were receiving Haldol, and 5 were receiving Stelazine. The schizophrenic group in Experiment II was comprised of 4 Haldol and 5 Stelazine patients. Subjects in Experiment III were receiving a variety of antipsychotic agents.

In addition, 10 Veteran's Administration outpatients receiving methadone also participated in the experiment. They were paid volunteer exheroin addicts from the Methadone Maintenance Outpatient Program and Total Abstinence Colony at Brentwood Veterans Administration Hospital. The median dose was 70 mg per day for these subjects, and they had been on the methadone program for a median of 7.5 months.

Controls were 12 nonprofessional staff members at Big Spring State Hospital. Six of these subjects were used in each of the first two experiments, these two groups being matched for age and education.

## Tasks

In all experiments visual displays on the screen of a graphics terminal were used to present subjects with four different tasks, graduated in terms of complexity. As can be seen from Figure 14.1, these tasks increased in difficulty; note the increased number of curvilinear relationships between cues and criteria from Task 1 through Task 4. In all tasks, however, an additive organizing principle was involved (see Chapter 3 for details).

These tasks were presented by two sets of stimulus materials; one (used in Experiments I and III) involved no substantive content, the other (used in Experiment II) using labels for both cues and criterion that made the task one of judging the quality of a "doctor."

### Experiment I

In the contentless investigation subjects were presented with 30 trials; on each trial the subject made a judgment regarding the values (which ranged from 1 to 20) of a

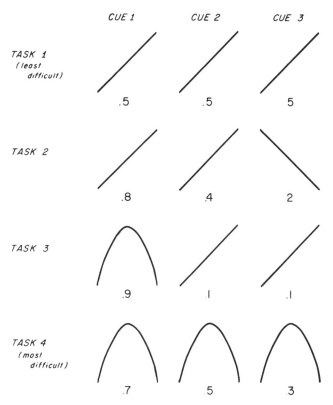

**Figure 14.1.**    Differential weights and function forms of tasks.

undefined criterion based on the values of three cues. Cue values (which ranged from 1 to 10) were presented by means of horizontal bars, the numerical value of the cue being represented by the length of the bar. No descriptive labels were attached to the cues.

## Experiment II

As in Experiment I, horizontal bars were used to present cue values. In this experiment, however, subjects were asked to judge "how good a doctor" an individual would be; each judgment was based on information given by cue values. The cues were an individual doctor's (1) intelligence, (2) interest in patients, and (3) age and experience in the medical profession. As in Experiment I, cue values ranged from 1 to 10 and criterion values from 1 to 20.

## Experiment III

As in the two experiments reported above, a three-cue task was used; cue values being presented by means of horizontal bars. In an effort to introduce more complexity into this task, all cues were related to the criterion in a curvilinear fashion, specifically as inverted-U functions. Cue-criterion correlations were set at .8, .4, and .2. As with those tasks used in Experiments I and II, the task contained irreducible uncertainty, $R^2$ (overall predictability) being .90.

## General Procedure

A Hazeltine 2000 visual interactive display console, connected by means of long distance telephone with a CDC 6400, was used to display the task materials and (in Experiments II and III) cognitive feedback. Subjects were seated before the console and cue values were presented on the screen (a cathode ray tube) of the console in the form of bar graphs as described above. Subjects entered their judgments directly into the central computer by means of the keyboard on the console.

Subjects were tested individually. Each subject was instructed that the purpose of the investigation was to determine how people learned to make judgments (in Experiments I and III how they learned to make numerical judgments, and in Experiment II judgments about the quality of doctors). They were then told that (a) they would be making judgments on the basis of certain items of information (cues); and (b) they would be given specific instructions concerning how to use this information to make such judgments accurately. The experimenter E presented a sample trial on the screen to demonstrate to the subject S the types of display S would be viewing. E then explained, in some detail, what was meant by cue weights, and illustrated specific cue-criterion functional relationships. S was next asked if he had questions and was required to repeat, in a general way, the instructions up to this point. S completed five "warm-up" trials during which E further clarified the nature of differential function forms and cue weights. These detailed instructions were intended to maximize knowledge of task parameters; cognitive control—the ability to implement knowledge—thereby becoming critical for performance.

S then completed the 15 experimental trials presented by means of the display apparatus. On all trials the level of each of the three cues was represented by a horizontal bar. S could thus gain information about cue values without performing any arithmetic calculations. S was allowed to view the display for a given trial for as long as he liked, although Ss, after the initial 10 or 15 trials, almost always responded within two minutes. *S* would enter his own response on the keyboard, after which the next trial would automatically be displayed on the screen.

## EXPERIMENT I

### Details of Procedure

Subjects from three groups—hospitalized chronic schizophrenics ($n$ = 11), methadone maintenance outpatients ($n$ = 10), and normal controls ($n$ = 6)—exercised their judgment with the four tasks described above.

Although control and methadone subjects completed all four tasks at a single sitting, the schizophrenic patients completed only one per session on each of four successive days. All subjects in the three groups completed all of the four experimental tasks; all subjects dealt with the tasks in the order from least (Task 1) to most (Task 4) complex.

As noted above, instructions in this study were geared to maximize knowledge, thus increasing the relative importance of control in accounting for drug-psychopathological group differences. The primary purpose of Experiment I, however, was to determine the utility of interactive computer graphics methods for use with difficult, generally poorly motivated, patients. If these patients could understand and make use of such displays (the criterion being effective performance), then further exploration of these procedures with similar populations would be justified.

### Results of Experiment I

#### *Achievement*

Adequacy of performance on judgment tasks is determined by correlating the subject's judgments with the correct values of the criterion. These achievement correlations $r_a$ were determined over 15 trials for each of the drug-pathology groups on each of the four learning tasks. As indicated in Figure 14.2, the order of group performance varies somewhat across tasks. Controls evidence the highest achievement on all four tasks, however, and the schizophrenics receiving antipsychotic drugs generally display the poorest achievement. A 4 × 3 analysis of variance (Task × Drug Group) yielded no statistically significant main effects or interactions.

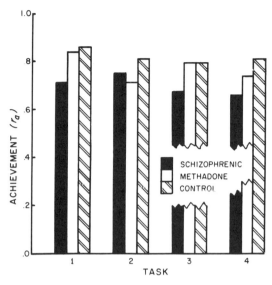

**Figure 14.2.**   Achievement $r_a$ of three drug-pathology groups under four task conditions increasing in complexity.

## Knowledge

Task knowledge $G$ measures the extent to which the subject has correctly detected properties of the task; that is, the extent to which a subject's cognitive system is isomorphic with the task system, independent of the uncertainty in both systems. As indicated in Figure 14.3, the relative performance of drug groups is the same over all four tasks and closely resembles the overall achievement results. That is, controls consistently perform better than the drug groups, with the schizophrenic drug group being the least effective group under *all* task complexity conditions. An ANOVA of $G$ results yielded a statistically significant main effect for drug groups ($F = 4.59$; $df = 2, 26$; $p < .05$).

## Cognitive Control

The measure of cognitive control is the multiple correlation $R$ between the cue values and a subject's responses over a series of trials. It is a measure of the predictability of the subject's response system (statistically independent of knowledge) and allows assessment of the extent to which the subject can effectively implement his knowledge. $R$ was determined over the complete 30 trials for each drug group and task condition. The results are summarized in Figure 14.4.

An ANOVA of these data yielded no statistically significant main effects or interactions. Each of the three groups performs best in at least one of the task

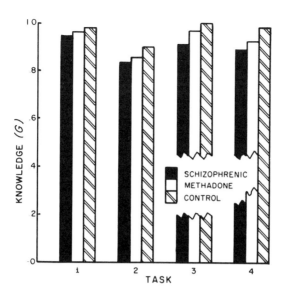

**Figure 14.3.** Knowledge $G$ in three drug-pathology groups under four task conditions increasing in complexity.

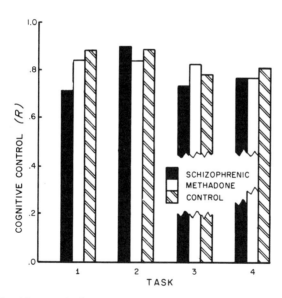

**Figure 14.4.** Cognitive control $R$ in three drug-pathology groups under four task conditions increasing in complexity.

conditions, although under no single task condition are the differences statistically significant.

Finally, there is some evidence that within the methadone group performance becomes increasingly dose dependent as task complexity increases. Dose level was a better predictor of achievement in Tasks 3 and 4 than age, IQ, education, or length of addiction to heroin or methadone; correlations between dose and achievement approached significance, $r = .60$ for Task 3 ($p < .10$) and .50 for Task 4. (The dose dependent effects of methadone are explored further by Weischselbaum in Chapter 15.)

## Conclusion

Results of the first investigation using interactive computer graphics techniques indicated that *(a)* the method was both understandable and motivating for even such traditionally difficult research subjects as chronic schizophrenics and drug addicts; *(b)* computer-assisted visual displays could be effectively utilized to evaluate psychopathological and drug influences; and *(c)* contrary to expectations, knowledge rather than control was the parameter most effected by drug-pathological group status.

Although it vindicated the appropriateness of using these techniques with such populations, the high level of achievement attained by all groups in the first experiment was surprising. These results suggest that computer-presented displays facilitate learning, even if used only for the presentation of task materials. On the other hand, such high achievement levels made it difficult to distinguish differences in drug influences; subjects perform well regardless of drug-psychopathology status.

In order to increase the discriminating capacity of the techniques, three courses of action were available. It would be possible to increase the complexity of the tasks either by increasing the number of cues to which a subject must attend, or by increasing the variety of functional relations between cues and criterion, or by increasing the complexity of the principle by which the cue data were combined. Where schizophrenic subjects are involved, however, the possibility of influencing level of achievement by adding *content* to the tasks should also be considered, since a number of studies have indicated that task content is critical to the cognitive performance of these patients. One investigation (Gillis, 1969) has demonstrated the impairing effects of interpersonal content on the judgmental learning performance of schizophrenics. Specifically, Gillis found that task content, which included social relevance, served to diminish achievement on tasks in which schizophrenic subjects had performed no differently than normals when *no content* was involved.

## EXPERIMENT II

In an attempt to discover whether similar negative effects on achievement levels would be found with the use of interactive computer graphics techniques, a study of the effects of *content* on the performance of schizophrenics was undertaken. This was accomplished by changing the description of the task to that of judging the "quality of a doctor" (as described in the method section). Again subjects were confronted with three cues, the values of which were represented by the lengths of bars. Again they made judgments on a criterion scale ranging from 1 to 20. In the "content" study, however, the criterion represented not an abstract number but "how good a doctor" an individual could be judged to be on the basis of cue values representing *(a)* his intelligence, *(b)* the extent of his interest in patients, and *(c)* his age/experience. The formal properties of the tasks remained the same.

On the assumption that the addition of content would depress the achievement levels of schizophrenic subjects, it was also decided to assess the consequences of *cognitive feedback*. This was accomplished by presenting subjects with two 15–trial blocks. After the first block subjects were presented with information concerning *(a)* the cue weights and function forms they employed on the first block of trials, and *(b)* a comparison of these cue-utilization strategies with actual task properties. It was expected that while overall performance of the schizophrenic group would be impaired (relative to Experiment I levels) by the addition of content to the tasks, the impairment would be mainly evident in the first (prefeedback) block of trials. Significant improvement would appear in the second block of trials, however, as a function of the cognitive feedback. Since normal controls (nonprofessional hospital staff) were not expected to evidence deterioration due to task content in block 1 it was expected that their performance would remain at a high level, but not necessarily show significant improvement, in block 2.

## Results of Experiment II

### *Effects of Task Content*

The critical questions in Experiment II concerned the importance of content and feedback. To evaluate the effects of content the performance of drug and control groups in Experiment II was compared with their performance on tasks having no content; that is, the tasks used in Experiment I. Because the contentless study (Experiment I) involved only 15 trials, performance here was compared with that in the first 15 trials of the interpersonal content (Experiment II) investigation.

Results of these comparisons are summarized for all four tasks in Figure 14.5. As may be seen, the performance of neither drug nor control subjects deteriorated greatly when content was included in the tasks. Control subjects generally maintained a performance level superior to schizophrenics and similar to the level they held in the contentless trials. Most important, the drug-schizophrenic group demonstrated no diminution as a function of task content. The only statistically significant differences obtained, in fact, were on the task variable, indicating that

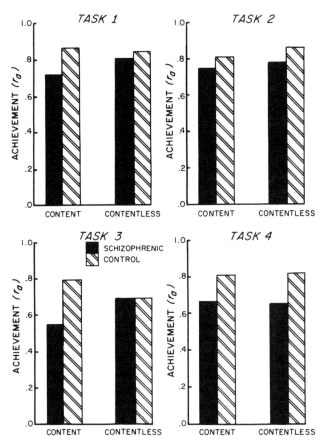

**Figure 14.5.**   Achievement $r_a$ of drug and control subjects under content and contentless task conditions.

performance for the combined groups deteriorated over the combined content and contentless trials as a function of increasing task complexity.

Results similar to those for achievement were obtained when knowledge $G$ and control $R$ were assessed separately. An analysis of variance (Task Complexity × Drug Groups × Content vs. Contentless Trials) of $G$ scores yielded a statistically significant main effect for drug group as had the contentless data (Experiment I). Analysis of cognitive control $R$ data yielded only a statistically significant main effect for task complexity, congruent with the overall achievement $r_a$ results.

*Effects of Feedback*

The primary advantage of the graphics techniques is that individuals are allowed to compare their *actual* manner of using information with the *intended* manner. Whereas this advantage has been demonstrated with samples of normals not receiving drugs, there are no data regarding the benefits of this type of feedback with psychopathological subjects. Experiment II provided an opportunity for investigating this problem. This was accomplished by giving subjects in both the schizophrenic and control samples feedback after the first 15 trials regarding *(a)* their own strategies of cue utilization, and *(b)* task properties. They then completed a second block of 15 trials in which such feedback could be implemented.

Performance was compared between the two 15-trial blocks in terms of overall achievement $r_a$ and its individual components $G$ and $R$. The results for achievement are described for all task conditions, and for both schizophrenic and control subjects in Figure 14.6. An analysis of variance of this achievement data (Group × Feedback Condition × Tasks) yielded no significant main effects or interactions. Similar analyses of $G$ and $R$ yielded only a significant main effect for group, controls' performance being significantly above that of schizophrenic subjects. Feedback, however, did not significantly improve the performance of either the schizophrenic or control groups in any of the four task conditions.

It is apparent, however, that circumstances did not allow an effective test of the utility of cognitive feedback. As considered above, performance on prefeedback trials was at such a high level that there was little room for improvement with any type of feedback. Therefore, it was decided to carry out a third study directed specifically at *comparing the effectiveness of different types of feedback for subjects receiving antipsychotic drugs.*

Before turning to Experiment III, however, the reader should take careful note that Experiment II confirmed the unexpected results of Experiment I and thereby provided very important information: schizophrenics (and normal) subjects have a far greater capacity for exercising control over their judgment than any research has ever demonstrated. This result, perhaps more than any other reported in this book, deserves careful study.

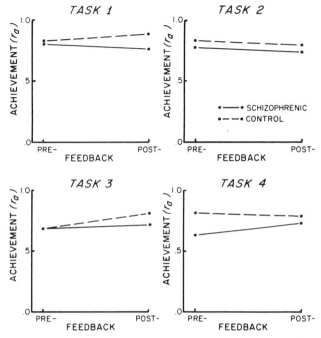

**Figure 14.6.**   Achievement $r_a$ of drug and control subjects in pre- and post-feedback conditions.

## EXPERIMENT III

The third investigation looked directly at the effects of different types of feedback on the ability of schizophrenic patients to learn to make social judgments. Three types of feedback were used—outcome, task feedforward, and cognitive feedback. Seventeen hospitalized schizophrenic patients, all receiving antipsychotic drugs, were randomly assigned to one of the feedback conditions. Subjects completed four blocks of twenty trials each on Task 4.

### Details of Feedback Conditions

In the outcome feedback condition, subjects were given the correct answer after they had made their judgment on each trial. In the task feedforward condition, subjects were given information about the structural properties of the task, that is, the cue-criterion correlations and function forms described above. This information was given *prior* to a subject's beginning the task and after each of the first three blocks of 20 trials. In the cognitive feedback condition subjects were given *both* the information regarding task properties *and* descriptions of their own cue-utilization strategies. Subjects, after each of the first three blocks of 20 trials, were shown visual displays of the actual cue weights and function forms and the weights and function forms they had employed over that block of trials. A subject could thus directly compare his judgmental strategy with the maximally effective strategy. These subjects were also given feedforward (task properties) prior to trial one, as in the feedforward condition. In presenting information regarding task characteristics prior to the first trial, conditions were again created that maximized the importance of cognitive control. Since subjects were provided with the task information essential to effective performance—and steps were taken to insure that they did understand this information—the principal difficulties with performance were likely to be caused by the problem of implementing such knowledge; that is, caused by the difficulties of cognitive control.

## Details of Procedure

Except for the differences necessitated by the feedback conditions, procedures were identical to those used in Experiments I and II. In order to assure that knowledge of task characteristics was maximized, the detailed explanation-demonstration-"practice trials" procedure described for Experiment I was again followed.

All subjects received 80 trials. On each trial, the three cues were presented as horizontal bars, the value of each cue being indicated by the length of the bar. No time limits were placed on subjects' observations of these cues. After arriving at a response, a subject entered his response on the terminal keyboard. In the outcome feedback condition, the correct answer was then displayed pictorially on the screen. Cue values for the next trial then appeared automatically. The sequence of events was the same for the feedforward and cognitive feedback conditions; no outcome feedback was provided in the latter two conditions.

## Results of Experiment III

### Achievement

Figure 14.7 describes achievement in the three feedback conditions over blocks of trials. An analysis of variance (Blocks $\times$ Feedback Groups) of these results

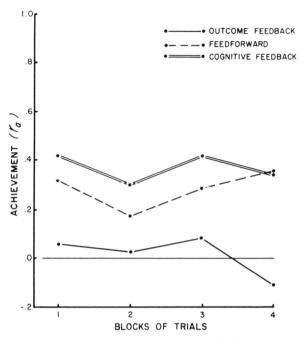

**Figure 14.7.** Achievement $r_a$ under three feedback conditions.

yielded a significant main effect for feedback conditions. While the feedforward and cognitive feedback groups demonstrate virtually identical achievement in the final block, the outcome feedback group is significantly inferior to these two; *actually showing a marked diminution in performance from its initial level.* The outcome group is, in fact, notably below the other feedback groups across all four blocks of trials, replicating with antipsychotic drug subjects the rather surprising results obtained with college students (Hammond, Summers, & Deane, 1973)—that outcome feedback actually *impairs* learning in judgmental learning situations.

The block 1 performance of the three groups also merits comment. Outcome feedback might not be expected to enhance learning during initial trials. The cue-criterion function forms were complex and subjects in this condition had received no prior information regarding such functional relationships or cue weights. Both the feedforward and cognitive feedback groups did receive such information, however, and made immediate use of it. These groups, in fact, did not improve performance over trials. The discrepancy between their achievement and that of the outcome feedback subjects increased, rather, as a function of the latter's deterioration in performance.

## Knowledge and Control

Since type of feedback does indeed exert a significant effect on performance, the important question is whether it accomplishes this by affecting knowledge or control (or both).

Figure 14.8 summarizes knowledge $G$ of the three feedback groups over trials. The feedforward and cognitive feedback groups, while similar to each other on this index, are superior to the outcome group in the initial trials (as anticipated) and maintain this superiority throughout the experimental trials. An analysis of variance of these knowledge results failed, however, to yield a significant main effect for feedback groups. What is perhaps most impressive about these findings is the deterioration of performance of the outcome feedback group. Although these subjects demonstrate some learning in the first two blocks of trials their knowledge scores thereafter decrease dramatically. Outcome feedback thus actually results in progressively *less* knowledge of task characteristics.

Results with regard to control $R^2$ yield much the same pattern (see Figure 14.9). The feedforward and cognitive feedback groups learn more rapidly than outcome subjects and maintain this advantage throughout the experimental trials. An

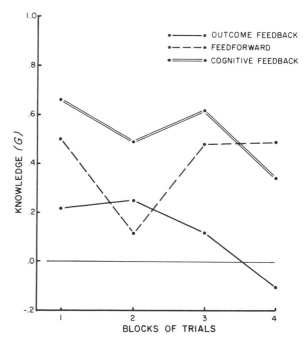

**Figure 14.8.** Knowledge $G$ under three feedback conditions.

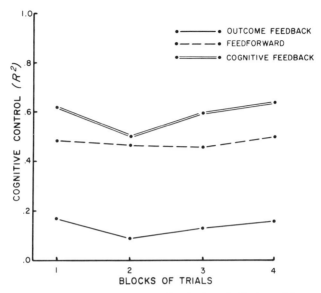

**Figure 14.9.**   Cognitive control $R^2$ under three feedback conditions.

analysis of variance performed on these control scores did, however, yield a significant main effect for feedback groups. *Feedback, that is, does make a difference in the ability of antipsychotic drug subjects to learn to make social judgments.* Although both the knowledge and control components of achievement are affected, significant differences are obtained only on the latter index. *Differences in performance are produced mainly as a result of the differential effects of different types of feedback on cognitive control.*

## SUMMARY AND DISCUSSION

Results from the three experiments lead to four primary conclusions: (1) interactive computer graphics techniques can be used with psychopathological populations and with individuals on a variety of chemotherapeutic regimens; (2) these methods appear to be sensitive to drug effects; (3) the type of feedback given, made possible by interactive computer graphics, is as critical for judgmental learning with drug-pathological groups as it is for normal college students; and (4) while both knowledge and control parameters are effected by an individual's drug-pathology status, feedback efficacy is primarily a function of the enhanced cognitive control induced by interactive computer graphics presentations.

Experiment I, the no-content, no-feedback study, yielded the following results: normal control subjects, receiving no psychoactive medication, performed best across tasks of varying levels of complexity. Schizophrenics on antipsychotic drug regimens were always least effective (although they did perform at a high level); methadone subjects performed at a level intermediate to these groups. Although this pattern of drug group differences reached statistical significance only for the knowledge component of achievement $G$, it was generally characteristic also of the control measure $R$ and the overall index of performance $r_a$. The results were, of course, not surprising given prior findings concerning impairment of complex learning by antipsychotic drugs (Gillis & Davis, 1973; Gillis, Chapters 4, 7, and 10, of this book). The most striking aspect of these data was, however, the *very high level of performance attained by all of the drug groups*, compared with past studies using similar tasks. To some extent this had been hoped for—the facilitation of learning was indeed the primary purpose for using the interactive computer graphics method with drug subjects—although it was somewhat surprising that this advantage could be so dramatically realized simply by using the device to present information.

Performance at such high levels for both drug and control groups created the possibility that drug influences on judgment were being masked. It was, therefore, necessary to take some steps to increase the complexity of the tasks.

Of the several possible methods of enhancing task complexity—for example, increasing the number of cues confronting subjects, or the difficulty of cue-criterion functional relationships—it was decided to investigate first the influence of task content on performance. It was expected that the addition of interpersonally relevant content to the tasks used in Experiment I would sufficiently diminish performance, and that differences between drug groups would become more apparent.

In addition, Experiment II sought to explore the effects of differential types of feedback on learning. Although evidence of the effectiveness of cognitive—as opposed to outcome—feedback existed for nonpsychiatric groups, use of these procedures had not yet been attempted for psychopathological patients or for groups receiving antipsychotic medications. By maintaining the same number of experimental trials (30) as in Experiment I, but presenting cognitive feedback between the two 15-trial blocks, Experiment II allowed an assessment of the utility of feedback.

Results suggested that neither the introduction of content nor feedback changes produced statistically significant effects. The performance of neither control nor drug-schizophrenic subjects was impaired by the interpersonal nature of the judgment task, nor was the achievement of either group facilitated by feedback.

This was true whether the indices involved were of overall achievement $r_a$ or of its individual components, knowledge $G$ and control $R$. Again the performance of controls was only slightly (though statistically significant) better than those of the patients.

The failure of feedback type or task content to make a significant difference was almost certainly due to the same "facilitation of learning" effects noted in Experiment I. Performance remained at such a high level under virtually all conditions that it was difficult to assess the consequences of content and feedback as well as differential drug effects.

Although this again established the motivating or attention-getting values of the computer terminal and the information it presents, it left the efficacy-of-feedback question untested. The issue is critical, however. Since any form of psychological treatment involves learning (Gillis, 1969, 1971), the question of effective feedback is vital to very practical problems of psychiatric treatment.

Experiment III was thus designed to investigate directly the relative efficacy of various forms of feedback. Results strongly substantiated the conclusions derived from studies of college students. Outcome feedback did indeed lead to increasingly *ineffective* performance; cognitive feedback and information regarding task structure were significantly more effective than outcome feedback.

It is somewhat premature to consider specific psychotherapeutic implications at this time, still, the general implications are clear; to the extent that ecological circumstances permit the kinds of structural descriptions and analyses of cognitive approach represented in our studies, feedback should be based on such analyses rather than on results. An obvious example will perhaps make the point. If a paranoid patient makes a judgment that another individual is hostile to him, it would be effective to analyze the specific cues (and weightings) he is using in arriving at such a conclusion and at least attempt to determine their actual ecological validities. Simply pointing out that he has often made similar judgments that have proved inaccurate will lead to little learning (that is, to little cognitive change in the way he approaches situations).

This possible application is directly tied to the feedback data. The more general results from this exploratory work with interactive computer graphics are those suggested at the outset of this section. They include the substantive findings that (a) even seriously ill psychiatric patients can be taught to make effective judgments when appropriate means of presenting stimuli and providing feedback are used; (b) type of feedback is critical to such learning; and (c) both knowledge and control parameters are affected. Interactive computer graphics techniques not only appear to facilitate learning, they also appear to be useful in research on the effects of drugs on the cognitive processes of patients.

The next steps in research of this type should include variations in task structures and complexity (much as was done in Experiment III) to make the method maximally sensitive to drug and psychopathological influences. It is also important that the interactive computer graphics method be integrated with the interpersonal learning approach described elsewhere in this book (for example, Gillis, Chapter 13). Since these methods enhance task learning (as results in all three of the studies reported here attest), it would be worth knowing how they affect socially mediated learning, more directly analogous to the traditional psychotherapeutic situation. The importance of determining differential drug effects, if any, on such therapy-relevant learning is apparent.

## REFERENCES

Gillis, J. S. Schizophrenic thinking in a probabilistic situation. *Psychological Record,* 1969, **19,** 211–224.

Gillis, J. S. Ecological relevance and the study of cognitive disorders. In J. Hellmuth (Ed.), *Cognitive studies II: Deficits in cognition.* New York: Brunner-Mazel, 1971.

Gillis, J. S. and Davis, K. E. The effects of psychoactive drugs on complex thinking in paranoid and nonparanoid schizophrenics: An application of the multiple-cue model to the study of disordered thinking. In L. Rappoport and D. Summers (Eds.), *Human judgment and social interaction.* New York: Holt, Rinehart & Winston, 1973.

Hammond, K. R. Computer graphics as an aid to learning. *Science,* 1971, **172,** 903–908.

Hammond, K. R. and Summers, D. A. Cognitive control. *Psychological Review,* 1972, **79,** 58–67.

Hammond, K. R., Summers, D. A., and Deane, D. H. Negative effects of outcome feedback in multiple-cue probability learning. *Organizational Behavior and Human Performance,* 1973, **9,** 30–34.

# CHAPTER 15

# New Concepts: Effects of Methadone Maintenance on Cognitive Control

HART F. WEICHSELBAUM

The rapid proliferation of methadone treatment centers throughout the United States has underscored the importance of investigating the effects of continued administration of maintenance dosages. Although methadone does provide a stable physiological milieu for those who have developed a tolerance for it, little research has been directed toward assessing the *cognitive* consequences of its prolonged use. As recently as 1973, Chambers, Brill, and Langrod stated, ". . . (we) are aware of *no* significant attempts to measure experimentally any cognitive impairment resulting from chronic administration of high doses of methadone [p. 170]."

Gritz, Jarvik, Dymond, Charuvastra, Shiffman, Haber, Coger, and Schlesinger (1974) have begun the task of assessing possible cognitive deficits in a methadone population. They administered a battery of tests measuring a variety of cognitive abilities to volunteer exheroin addicts receiving methadone and to control subjects, and found that only the most complex tests of learning and immediate recall differentiated between the groups; simpler tests of learning and attention did not.

As indicated throughout this book, the ability to use information effectively to make accurate inferences or to draw conclusions correctly is important; those who cannot exercise their judgment well do not fare well in society. Therefore it is of some importance to determine whether methadone addicts suffer a deficit in this regard. Gillis, Stewart, and Gritz (see Chapter 14) took the first steps in this direction. They found that knowledge and control in judgment tasks were only slightly impaired for addicts on methadone maintenance treatment (as was also the case with schizophrenics receiving antipsychotic medication) compared to a group of normal control subjects. Their results paralleled those obtained (Gritz et al.,

1974) with regard to other tests of cognitive functioning. In addition, Gillis and colleagues (Chapter 14) found an indication that the performance of the methadone group might be *dose-dependent* for the more complex tasks: dose level was a better predictor of achievement in their judgment tasks than age, IQ, education, or length of addiction to methadone or heroin. As a result of this finding, the general aim of the present study (part of a larger investigation reported elsewhere, Weichselbaum, 1974) was to compare the performance of addict and nonaddict groups on three judgment tasks differing in complexity.

More specifically, the present study was concerned with the ability of methadone addicts to exercise *cognitive control*, that is, exercise their judgment in a specific way. As in the study reported in Chapter 14, methadone addicts were asked to arrive at a judgment by assigning specific weights and function forms to a set of cues. The present study was, therefore, similar to the experiment described by Gillis, Stewart, and Gritz but there were two important differences:

1. Drug-free inmates of a county jail, incarcerated for at least two weeks before their participation in the study, served as a control group, instead of hospital staff members as in the Gillis study. In the present study the use of similar narcotic-dependent and narcotic-free groups, whose drug use in the immediate past could be known with some certainty, permitted a more accurate assessment of drug-related differences in performance.

2. The range of task difficulty was increased. Very high levels of achievement and control in the Chapter 14 study suggested a ceiling effect for performance in their study. It was expected that increased task complexity would accentuate drug-related impairment of performance.

## METHOD

### Subjects

A total of 36 subjects participated in the study. The experimental group consisted of 24 ambulatory methadone patients receiving between 30 and 100 mg (oral) of methadone daily through a local, federally licensed polydrug clinic. Interviews revealed that subjects in the experimental group used a variety of licit and illicit drugs in the six months prior to their participation, although without exception they reported an opiate as their drug of choice. All subjects in the group had been receiving methadone daily for a minimum of four months.

Subjects in the methadone group were asked to abstain from using drugs other than methadone for 24 hours preceding an experimental session. There was evidence that most (19 of 24) complied: results from a weekly urinalysis conducted as part of the clinic program generally corroborated the addicts' self-reports.*

The control group consisted of individuals with social histories and demographic characteristics approximating those of the addicts. Twelve county jail inmates who were drug-free for two weeks preceding the experiment agreed to participate in the study. None had ever been addicted to narcotics, though seven had had an opportunity to try heroin, and two had actually used the drug for short periods of time.

**Table 15.1.   Comparison of Methadone and Control Groups**

| Variable | Methadone Group | | Control Group | |
|---|---|---|---|---|
| | Mean | Standard Deviation | Mean | Standard Deviation |
| Age | 24.4 | 2.57 | 25.2 | 3.79 |
| Marital status (1 = single, 2 = married) | 1.4 | .50 | 1.6 | .51 |
| Education (grade completed) | 11.9 | 1.56 | 12.0 | 1.54 |
| Father's socioeconomic status[a] | 5.0 | 1.35 | 4.9 | 1.16 |
| Length of heroin use (yrs.) | 5.4 | 2.81 | – | – |
| Length of methadone use (mos.) | 20.1 | 14.25 | – | – |
| Dose level | 57.3 | 22.36 | – | – |

[a]This score represents the occupational component of Hollingshead's Two Factor Index of Socioeconomic Status and is determined by having subject choose from 14 categories describing father's occupation. Scores range from 1 (low status) to 7 (high status).

Table 15.1 presents the demographic data for the two groups. In general, the control and experimental groups were comparable on a number of dimensions including sex and racial composition (predominantly white males), age (between 20 and 30), educational level attained (about twelfth grade), marital status (roughly half were married), and father's socioeconomic status (predominantly middle class). Subjects in both groups were volunteers, were cooperative through all phases of the study, and were paid $15 for their participation.

*An observed urine sample is collected from each methadone patient by the clinic staff at least once a week on a random basis. The urinalysis procedure can detect amphetamines, barbiturates, cocaine, codeine, methadone, morphine, and a variety of "unknown" substances, but not marijuana or alcohol. Nineteen of the 24 subjects had clean urine samples (i.e., no drugs present) for the two weeks preceding the experiments, while five had used morphine, cocaine, or barbiturates.

## Tasks

The weights and function forms of the three judgment tasks are presented in Figure 15.1. The cue-criterion correlations were .8, .4, and .2 in each task; the intercorrelations among the cues did not exceed .05. Cue values ranged from 1 to 10 and criterion values from 1 to 20. Task complexity was varied by using a different combination of function forms for each task. Since linear function forms are easier to learn than nonlinear function forms (Brehmer, 1970; Hammond & Summers, 1965) and positive function forms are easier to learn than negative function forms (Bjorkman, 1965; Naylor & Clark, 1968), the order of presumed task complexity, from least to most complex, was: Task 1 (three positive linear function forms), Task 2 (three inverted U-shaped function forms), and Task 3 (one negative linear, one U-shaped, and one inverted U-shaped function form). A general description of this research paradigm may be found in Chapter 3.

## Procedure

Each subject completed all three 20-trial tasks, yielding a 2 (Drug Conditions) × 3 (Task Complexity) factorial design with repeated measures on the second factor. The order of presentation of the tasks was varied over the three experimental sessions to counterbalance order effects.

Subjects received detailed instruction in "learning how another person makes judgments." Although the task was contentless (i.e., the cues lacked descriptive labels), the judgment process of a baseball team manager evaluating a prospective player was used to illustrate the application of weights and function forms. The subject was told that the cue values might represent scores on three aspects of a player's ability, for example, hitting, running, and fielding. Cue weights describe the relative importance of the cue to the criterion, and function forms indicate the functional relationship between cue and criterion. In each trial, the subject was asked to make a judgment about the numerical value of an unobserved criterion on the basis of the values of the three cues. Unlike the procedure in Chapter 14, the instructions emphasized understanding the meaning of the task parameters rather than policy execution. Sample trials were provided to ensure that the subject understood the task, but he was given no prior experience with any of the tasks used in the study.

At the beginning of each session, the subject was given a task description sheet with the properties of the task to be learned, that is, the cue-criterion correlations

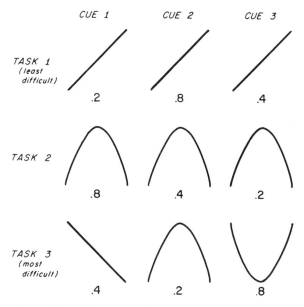

**Figure 15.1.**   Differential weights and function forms of tasks.

(weights) and function forms for each cue. The interactive computer graphics procedure described in Chapter 14 was used to present task materials, and the subject completed each 20-trial task at his own pace.

All subjects completed the tasks in three half-hour sessions, with no more than two sessions on a single day to minimize the effects of fatigue. Subjects in the methadone group participated in the study between 2 and 6 hours after receiving their daily medication so that drug effects would be fairly constant across the group.

## RESULTS

Performance was assessed in terms of the accuracy of the subject's judgments (achievement), the extent to which he acquired information about task properties (knowledge), and the consistency with which he applied this information (control). The three indices were computed for each subject, transformed into Fisher's $z$-scores, and entered into a 2 (Drug Conditions) × 3 (Task Complexity) analysis of variance with repeated measures on the last factor.

## Achievement

The ANOVA indicated that achievement (the correlation between the criterion values and subject's responses) varied with task complexity, $F = 21.37$; $df = 2$, $34$; $p < .01$. As expected, mean $r_a$ decreased from Task 1 to Task 3. Figure 15.2 illustrates quite clearly that the presumed order of difficulty was correct.

Although the mean achievement $r_a$ of the control group was slightly better than that of the methadone group (.93 vs. .91), the difference was far from significant; the performance of the two groups was essentially identical.

## Knowledge and Control

The effect of task complexity on achievement is clarified by an examination of its component measures, *(a)* knowledge (the correlation between the least squares prediction of subject's responses from the cues and the least squares prediction of the criterion values from the cues) and *(b)* control (the multiple correlation between the cue values and the subject's responses). An ANOVA performed with these indices revealed main effects of task complexity on $G$ ($F = 16.58$; $df = 2$,

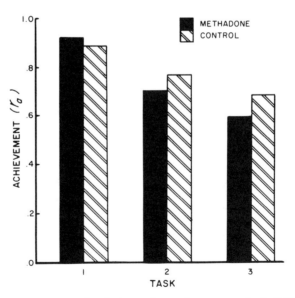

**Figure 15.2.** Achievement $r_a$ of methadone and control groups over the three tasks.

34; $p < .01$), and on $R^2$ ($F = 13.58$; $df = 2, 34$; $p < .01$). Thus the subject's knowledge of how information should be utilized as well as his capacity to implement that knowledge were affected by task complexity, and both contributed to the diminution of achievement across tasks.

There were no significant differences between the methadone and control groups, however. Again, the performance of these groups was essentially the same (see Figures 15.3 and 15.4).

## Correlations between Dose Level and Performance Measures

The finding (Gillis, et al.) that performance on complex inference tasks tended to be dose-dependent for 10 methadone subjects suggested the possibility that daily dose level is a more meaningful variable than methadone use per se in assessing drug-related effects. An analysis that takes into account the amount of methadone each subject was receiving might detect measurable cognitive effects obscured by a gross comparison of group mean achievement.

Correlation coefficients between dose level and performance measures for the 24 drug-dependent subjects were computed and revealed that dose and achieve-

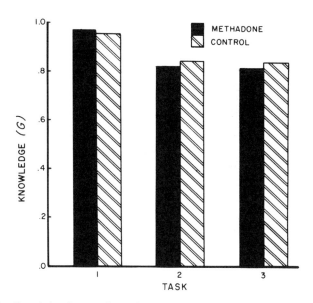

**Figure 15.3.** Knowledge $G$ scores for methadone and control groups over the three tasks.

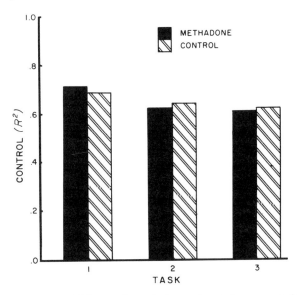

**Figure 15.4.**    Cognitive control $R^2$ scores for methadone and control groups over the three tasks.

ment were indeed inversely related for the most complex task ($r = -.48; p < .05$; $r_a$ transformed to Fisher $z$-scores). A scatter plot of this relationship appears in Figure 15.5. Both knowledge ($r = .52; p < .05; G$ transformed to Fisher $z$-scores) and control $R^2$ ($r = -.42; p < .05$) contributed to the negative association.

## DISCUSSION

The results regarding drug-related impairment of cognitive functioning supported earlier findings (Gritz et al., 1974; and Gillis et al., Chapter 14); there was essentially no difference in the mean performance of the addict group as compared to the control group. Also, the finding by Gillis and colleagues that higher dosages of methadone tended to be associated with performance deficits for difficult inference tasks was substantiated.

The fact that this relationship has been found to hold for 34 patients in two treatment programs gains significance because it bears directly on an issue of considerable clinical interest. A controversy currently exists within the treatment field concerning the relative efficacy of high versus low dose maintenance therapy (see, for example, Bowling, Moffett, & Taylor, 1973; Brill, 1973). Recent research has indicated that patients on low doses (below 50 mg) do as well in

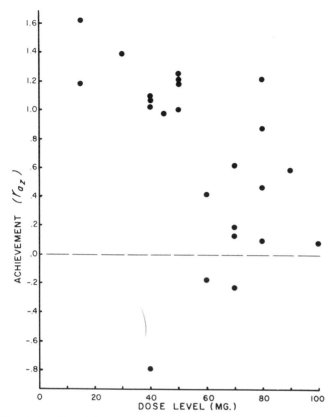

**Figure 15.5.**   A plot of the relation between methadone dose level and achievement $r_{a_z}$ for Task 3 (n = 24).

achieving treatment goals as those on high (above 70 mg) doses (Bowling et al., 1973) and experience fewer somatic side effects, such as dermatitis, constipation, and impotence (Goldstein, 1970). Clearly, if, as the present results suggest, cognitive impairment can be added to the list of undesirable side effects that are dose-related, the case for low dose maintenance becomes more compelling.

The inadequacies of the present design are quite apparent; studies involving double-blind and concurrent assignment to dosage groups are required to eliminate competing explanations of the results. The present study clearly shows, however, that the judgmental learning methodology provides a context in which this investigation can be conducted.

Finally, it is important to note that the cognitive capabilities of human subjects have been underestimated. Very high levels of achievement for both the addict and the inmate groups provide further evidence that cognitively oriented task information makes it possible to exercise considerable control over one's judgment, and thus to learn extremely complex inference tasks. Consequently, further changes in the structure and complexity of judgment tasks are necessary to detect consistent and reliable drug-related effects, if, indeed, such drug-related effects exist.

## REFERENCES

Bjorkman, M. Learning of linear functions: Comparisons between a positive and a negative slope. Psychological Laboratories of the University of Stockholm, Report No. 183, 1965.

Bowling, C. E., Moffett, A. D., and Taylor, W. High versus low-dose maintenance therapy: An empirical test. In C. D. Chambers and L. Brill (Eds.), *Methadone: Experiences and issues*. New York: Behavioral Publications, 1973.

Brehmer, B. Inference behavior in a situation where the cues are not reliably received. *Organizational Behavior and Human Performance*, 1970, **5**, 330–347.

Brill, L. High versus low-dose maintenance therapy: A review of program experiences. In C. D. Chambers and L. Brill (Eds.), *Methadone: Experiences and issues*. New York: Behavioral Publications, 1973.

Chambers, C. D., Brill, L., and Langrod, J. Physiological and psychological side effects reported during maintenance therapy. In C. D. Chambers and L. Brill (Eds.), *Methadone: Experiences and issues*. New York: Behavioral Publications, 1973.

Goldstein, A. Blind controlled dosage comparisons with methadone in 200 patients. *Proceedings of the Third National Methadone Conference*. U. S. Public Health Service No. 2172, Rockville, Md.: National Institute of Mental Health, 1970.

Gritz, E. R., Jarvik, M. E., Dymond, A. M., Charuvastra, V. C., Shiffman, S. M. Haber, J., Coger, R., and Schlesinger, J. Physiological and psychological effects of methadone in man. Unpublished manuscript, Los Angeles, Brentwood Veterans Administration Hospital, 1974.

Hammond, K. R. and Summers, D. A. Cognitive dependence on linear and nonlinear cues. *Psychological Review*, 1965, **72**, 215–234.

Naylor, J. D. and Clark, R. D. Intuitive inference strategies in interval learning tasks as a function of validity magnitude and sign. *Organizational Behavior and Human Performance*, 1968, **3**, 378–399.

Weichselbaum, H. F. The effects of methadone maintenance on task learning with feedforward and cognitive feedback. University of Colorado Institute of Behavioral Science, Program of Research on Human Judgment and Social Interaction, Report 174, 1974.

# CHAPTER 16

# New Analyses: Application of Judgment Theory to Physicians' Judgments of Drug Effects

THOMAS R. STEWART, C. R. B. JOYCE, and MICHAEL K. LINDELL

All drugs purporting to be therapeutic must eventually be tried in human beings. This is usually first done by giving low single doses to a small number of healthy people. This step can, of course, demonstrate only that it is safe to give the substance to man, not that it is effective. If this step is passed satisfactorily, the potential drug is given to a small sample of patients suffering from relevant diseases. Unless it is a drug with effects as dramatic as those of penicillin, especially in diseases previously difficult to treat, too little will still be known at this stage about its profile of actions to obtain more than indications of its promise. It will soon have to be tried upon a larger sample in order to define more exactly the kind of patient for whom it is expected to be useful.

The principles of experimental design and statistical analysis that must be used in such "clinical trials" are those employed in other biological sciences and do not need to be explained here. The essential point is that the conditions hold while the investigation is carried out. That is, the conditions should be so controlled that results from each patient can be validly compared, and that any genuine effect of the drug can be reliably detected. As many sources of error may obscure the fact that the drug is of value, the appropriate procedure is to first identify such sources, remove those that can be removed, reduce those that cannot be eliminated entirely, hold constant those that can be controlled and, finally, estimate the magnitude of those that remain. The analysis of variance (ANOVA) is frequently used for this purpose. With an appropriate design, the effects of the new drug (in comparison with the old remedy, or a placebo) upon the variables being measured can be separated from effects due to differences between patients being studied, or to differences in the response of the same patient observed at different times. It may also be possible to distinguish between different groups of patients on the basis of their response, and then, post hoc, to look for explanations; or, as will need to be done in any case, to set up and examine the effects upon groups differing in defined relevant ways.

But whatever the details of the experimental design, the evaluation of the effect of a given treatment on a given patient is commonly left to the judgment of a physician. It is only on rare occasions that differences between participating physicians (if more than one is involved) or other judges are looked at; and possible changes in the behavior of a single judge over time are almost never looked for at all. This may be due to the frequent assumption (not only by laymen) that the training of the physician results in such a reliable and objective performance that no account need be taken of variation from this source; and also, because methods for handling the problem have not been readily available until recently. Until now, this source of error has at best been controlled, to an uncertain extent, by holding discussions between the participants before and perhaps during the trial. It is invariably lumped in with residual error (which, of course, it inflates), and so the likelihood of demonstrating a significant drug effect is reduced. Even if statistical significance is neglected in favor of clinical importance, the problem remains.

The implications are even more serious when, as is more and more frequently the case today, it becomes necessary for a variety of reasons (pressure of time, demands of national drug regulatory authorities, comparative rarity of the disease in the practice of any one physician) to resort to so-called *multicenter* clinical trials, which may even involve the participation of doctors from more than one country, having potentially very different medical training and background. It is clear that the problem needs attention, and a solution is proposed in this chapter.

A clinical trial may be of any degree of complexity. The investigator may have only to measure the blood pressure before and after the administration of an antihypertensive drug on one occasion and placebo on another, or he may study 30 or 40 different measures of clinical response, measured weekly for a period of six months or five years. These measures provide a detailed record of the time course of physiological or psychological changes relevant to the course of the disease or the action of the drug, and they—or a selection of them perhaps combined or transformed in some way—enable the physician to decide whether the treatment received by each patient was successful. Although the detailed analysis is important, the physician's overall judgment represents the best estimate of the treatment's probable utility to the individual patient. A set of such judgments is the best estimate of its value in general use.

Now each of these summary evaluations is a compound of the values that each physician has placed upon the clinical measures. These may differ from patient to patient, treatment to treatment, and occasion to occasion, and certainly from physician to physician. Even if the likelihood of such differences has been recognized and discussed at the outset, and agreement reached in principle about the way in which each element is to be entered into the overall judgment, it would clearly be desirable to have a method of monitoring the trial as it progresses to ensure that consistency is maintained between and within physicians.

An approach similar to that used in the different contexts described in preceding chapters enables this to be done. This chapter includes a brief statement of the theory of decision error in statistical testing followed by a description of the theory applied to clinical trials. The use of judgment policy analysis to permit improved precision of statistical tests and to isolate components of variation due to inconsistency of judges, differences among judges, differences among patients, and treatment differences is then discussed and illustrated. Since some of the statistical theory contained in this chapter is technical and only summarized briefly, the reader may wish to consult a statistical text (for example, Bailey, 1971, Chapters 14 and 15) for further explanation.

## THEORY

The notion of a decision error is basic to the theory of statistical testing. A decision error occurs when, in the course of testing the validity of a hypothesis about a distribution function, the investigator rejects a hypothesis when it is, in fact, correct.

There are two types of decision error: an error of the first kind, the Type I error, occurs when the null (no difference) hypothesis $H_0$ is falsely rejected; an error of the second kind, or Type II error, is made when the alternative hypothesis $H_A$ is falsely rejected. A contingency table shows these errors and their probabilities (see Table 16.1). The probability of correctly rejecting a null hypothesis (such as the difference between two means, $\mu_1 - \mu_2 = 0$) is of particular interest to the

**Table 16.1.   The Decision Model**

|  | State of Nature | |
| --- | --- | --- |
| Action | $H_0$ True | $H_A$ True |
| Reject $H_0$ | Type I $(\alpha)$ | Correct $(\pi)$ |
| Reject $H_A$ | Correct | Type II $(\beta)$ |

researcher. This probability $[\pi = 1 - \beta]$ is referred to as the *power* of the test to reject the null hypothesis correctly. For fixed $\alpha$, power increases as sample size $n$ increases. Given a specific alternative hypothesis (such as $\mu_1 - \mu_2 = \Delta$, where $\Delta$ has some specific value), a probability $\alpha$ and the sample size $n$, one can compute the power of the test $\pi$ or its complement $\beta$. Though valuable in post hoc analyses of experiments, statistical power analysis can be used most effectively in the *design* of experiments. Given desired protection levels against Type I and Type II errors and a specific alternative hypothesis $(H_A: \mu_1 - \mu_2 = \Delta)$, an appropriate sample size can be computed. Use of the sample size determined in this way ensures a fair test of $H_0$ against $H_A$. An illustration of the application of these principles follows.

## APPLICATION

Seven physicians, representing seven trial centers, based their judgment of the therapeutic effectiveness of a new mild analgesic drug on patients' reports of pain level at five intervals after application of the treatment. Investigators' judgments were entered on individual patient record sheets as a numerical rating between 1 (no therapeutic effectiveness) and 4 (complete therapeutic effectiveness). Six drug treatments were used. The treatments used by each investigator and the number of patients he treated differed (Table 16.2). For the first two examples, only the observations made by one physician on two drugs are used (treatment numbers 3 and 6). There were 60 patients; 30 received each treatment. Since the principles of statistical power analysis are the same for both ANOVA and $t$-test, the latter has been used to simplify the explanation. Although the distribution of the observa-

**Table 16.2.    Number of Patients Administered Each Treatment by Each Investigator**

| Treatment | \multicolumn{7}{c}{Investigator} | Totals |
|---|---|---|---|---|---|---|---|---|
|  | 1 | 2 | 3 | 4 | 5 | 6 | 7 |  |
| 1 |  | 25 | 16 |  | 25 |  |  | 66 |
| 2 | 30 |  |  | 16 | 25 | 10 | 20 | 101 |
| 3 | 30 | 25 | 16 | 16 | 25 | 10 | 23 | 145 |
| 4 |  |  |  |  |  |  | 23 | 23 |
| 5 |  | 25 | 16 |  | 25 |  |  | 66 |
| 6 | 30 |  |  | 16 |  | 10 |  | 56 |
| Totals | 90 | 75 | 48 | 48 | 100 | 30 | 66 |  |

tions is only approximately normal (due to the discrete nature of the dependent variable), the effect of this violation is probably minimal, because the sample variances are nearly equal and sample sizes are the same.

## A POSTERIORI DESIGN ANALYSIS

Consider the data in the example below.

**Example 1**

| Mean Efficacy Judgment | Standard Deviation | $n$ |
|---|---|---|
| $M_6 = 3.30$ | $\hat{S}_6 = 1.02$ | 30 |
| $M_3 = 3.07$ | $\hat{S}_3 = 1.12$ | 30 |

$$t = \frac{M_6 - M_3}{[S_{(M_6 - M_3)}]} = \frac{.23}{.281} \quad p > .05; \quad \text{nonsignificant}$$

*Postanalysis $A_1$*

Let us set $\alpha = .05$, $\beta = .05$. Since $n = 60$, fixing $\alpha = .05$, $\beta = .05$ defines an alternative hypothesis $H_{\tilde{A}}$: that $\mu_6 - \mu_3 \geqslant .65$. Under these conditions, then, we have implicitly decided that the smallest difference $\Delta$ that is worth detecting is three times as large as the obtained difference, $M_6 - M_3 = .23$.

*Postanalysis $A_2$*

Set $\alpha = .01$, $\beta = .01$. For this more stringent test the implicit alternative hypothesis is $H_{\tilde{A}}$: $\mu_6 - \mu_3 = .92$. This difference is substantial—four times as large as the obtained difference, and approximately 30% of the range (1–4) of the response scale.

*Postanalysis B*

Suppose that the obtained difference, $M_6 - M_3$, is true for the population (i.e., $\mu_6 - \mu_3 = .23$) and is a clinically important difference. The probability of falsely rejecting this difference, given the sample size in this experiment and $\alpha = .05$, is $\beta$

= .70. In other words, we would expect that 70% of the independent replications of this test would (incorrectly) fail to reject the hypothesis of no difference. Given the actual sample size and setting $\alpha = .01$ leads to $\beta \approx 1.00$. In short, with $N = 60$, $\alpha = .01$; $\mu_6 - \mu_3 = .23$, the investigator will almost certainly be unable to reject the alternative hypothesis, thus making the trial virtually useless.

## A Priori Design Analysis

If we wish to design an experiment that will detect a true (population) difference $\mu_6 - \mu_3 = .23$, with error probabilities $\alpha = .05, \beta = .05$, the $N$ required is 292 ($n_1 = n_2 = 146$; half being given each treatment). For $\alpha = .01, \beta = .01$, we need an $N = 546$.

The conclusion to be drawn from these sample sizes is clear. To detect a small but clinically important difference under the above circumstances a very large sample is required, much larger than was used in the trials conducted at each center in the present study. If the power of the experiment described could be improved only by increasing sample size, the investigator would be faced with a long, tedious and perhaps expensive experiment. But since the power function of the $t$-test is based upon the noncentrality parameter:

$$\phi = \frac{\mu_6 - \mu_3}{\sigma_e} \left(\frac{N}{2}\right)^{1/2}$$

the power of the experiment can be improved by reducing the estimate of the population variance ($\sigma_e^2$) instead of increasing sample size. Since our dependent variable is a *judgment* of effectiveness, consideration of judgment theory will indicate how this can be accomplished.

As already briefly outlined, the physician attends to a number of different cues in forming an appraisal of the overall effectiveness of a drug. These cues represent some of the larger number of different effects that the drug could have on a patient. *Physicians will be less than perfectly reliable in combining these cues and making their judgments.* Due to the complexity of the judgment task, the physician will be able to maintain only imperfect cognitive control over the execution of his judgmental policy. Thus he will tend to add error variance or "noise" to the systematic variance in his judgments. Physicians will also differ among themselves in the weights they attach to the cues. For instance, some will attribute more importance to early changes while other physicians may feel that a definite change at 4 hours is most important. Either may be correct, or both, or neither. In any case the resulting judgments will be less appropriate than they could have been. Effects of each of these phenomena upon the statistical test are discussed in turn. (See Chapter 3 for a description of judgment theory.)

## Imperfect Cognitive Control

The addition of a "noise" component to the systematic judgmental variance will decrease the power of any test using a judgment as a dependent variable. Conversely, removal of "noise" increases the power of a statistical test. The magnitude of this random component can be estimated by $\sqrt{1-R_s^2}$, where $R_s^2$ is the squared multiple correlation coefficient obtained from regressing the physician's judgments on the cues. Removal of the error component leaves only the predictable portion of the response variance ($s_{\hat{Y}_s}^2$)—rather than the total response variance ($s_{Y_s}^2$)—as an estimate of the population variance $\sigma^2$. Since $s_{\hat{Y}_s}^2 = R_s^2 s_{Y_s}^2$ and $0.0 \leqslant R_s^2 \leqslant 1.0$, use of only the predictable portion of the response variance ($s_{\hat{Y}_s}$) as an estimate of $\sigma^2$ will, for given protection levels ($\alpha,\beta$) and a specific alternative hypothesis $(H_A)$, require a smaller sample size than will use of the estimate ($s_{Y_s}^2$).

## Example 2

The design analysis section of Example 1 showed that, with $H_A : \mu_6 - \mu_3 = .23$, protection levels ($\alpha, \beta = .05$) required $n_1 = n_2 = 146$ and for ($\alpha, \beta = .01$), $n_1 = n_2 = 273$. The effectiveness of using $\hat{s}_{\hat{Y}_s}$ instead of $\hat{s}_{Y_s}$ ($= 1.08$) in the reduction of required sample size is shown for high ($R = .90$) and low ($R = .70$) levels of linear consistency (see Table 16.3). In short, when $R = .70$ use of the predictable portion of the judgment ($\hat{Y}_s$) rather than judgments ($Y_s$) themselves permits the investigator to cut sample size *in half*. Thus, the less reliable the judge the smaller the sample required, when his judgments are replaced by those derived from his policy equation.

Table 16.3.   Required Sample Sizes for Various Levels of $R$, $\alpha$, and $\beta$

| $R$ | $\alpha, \beta$ | $n_1, n_2$ |
| --- | --- | --- |
| 1.00 | .05 | 146 |
| .90 | .05 | 115 |
| .70 | .05 | 70 |
| 1.00 | .01 | 273 |
| .90 | .01 | 215 |
| .70 | .01 | 130 |

## Differences between Physicians

The statistical effects of differences in the judgmental policies of physicians can best be understood in terms of the ability of their policies to discriminate between two drugs. Assume, as in the example above, that the task involves the evaluation of the effectiveness of two drugs. Let us suppose further that a number of physicians make (independent) judgments of effectiveness and that these ratings are based on the same patients. In general, it will turn out that for some physicians (Group A) a $t$-test for Drug 1 versus Drug 2 will be significant and for others (Group B) the test will be nonsignificant. Since Groups A and B both judged the same patients, we can conclude that differences as to whether or not to reject $H_0$ occurred because the former group put higher weights ($\beta_{s_i}$) on those cues ($X_i$) on which the two drug groups differed most. The latter group of physicians put high weights on those cues on which the drug groups differed *least* (that is $\beta_{s_i}$ was high on those cues for which $X_{i_1} - X_{i_2}$ was small).

The fact that different judgmental policies produce different test results when applied to the *same* set of patients indicates that the solution of the problem is likely to be even more difficult when applying different policies to *different* sets of patients. In the latter case, we do not know whether it is differences in the physicians' judgmental policies or lack of generality in the drug effects that causes failures in replication between physicians. The net effect of the differences between physicians will be inadequate power of a statistical test to discriminate all but the most substantial differences in drug effects. In other words, since the power of the test against a modest difference ($H_A$: $\mu_1 - \mu_2 = \Delta$, where $\Delta$ is small) is too low, too often it will be concluded that a new drug is not efficacious when in fact it is. The same will be true for judgments about tolerability.

The problem of multiple judgment policies may be resolved by generalizing the solution to the problem of imperfect cognitive control. There the single physician was replaced by a mathematical model of his judgmental policy. Here a variety of policies is replaced by one model. This situation is considered next, and is illustrated by application to real-trial observations.

## Example 3

In this example the cues for the judgment were the patients' reports at five time intervals after treatment. Since it is likely that the investigators considered patterns in the patients' reports, five more cues, each based on such a possible pattern, discerned by one of the present authors and a colleague, were generated (Table 16.4). A total of 10 variables (five direct-report cues and five pattern cues) were used in the multiple regression analysis to predict each physician's judgments. The squared multiple correlations indicate the fit of the model based on the 10 variables to each investigator's judgments (Table 16.4). All the squared multiple correlations are statistically significant and are similar in magnitude to those observed in other studies of judgmental policy (Slovic & Lichtenstein, 1973, review such studies). For six of the seven investigators, the squared multiple correlations approach the limits of the reliability of human judgmental systems, thus suggesting that nearly all the reliable variation in the judgments of these investigators has been "captured" by the analysis. The seventh investigator ($\#5, R^2 = .489$) may be more unreliable than the other investigators; or he may be using cues not represented among the 10 variables included in the analysis; or he may have changed his judgmental system during the trial. Procedures for discriminating among these alternatives are available (Smith, 1972) but are beyond the scope of this chapter. For purposes of illustration, we treat this investigator as we have treated the others, and assume that the regression analysis has captured the reliable judgment policies controlling each investigator's judgments.

In Table 16.4 the weights for each investigator indicate the relative importance he attached to each cue. There are important differences among the investigators. The cue most highly weighted by one investigator is often ignored by another. Such differences in judgmental weighting systems are likely to produce different

**Table 16.4.  Beta Weights Produced by Judgmental Policy Analysis**

| Cues | Investigator | | | | | | |
|---|---|---|---|---|---|---|---|
| | 1 | 2 | 3 | 4 | 5 | 6 | 7 |
| Time of pain reports | | | | | | | |
| 0 hour | −.002 | .131 | .054 | −.111 | −.114 | −.275 | .825 |
| 1/2 hour | .025 | .233 | .266 | .317 | .634 | .058 | −.226 |
| 1 hour | −.041 | .224 | −.298 | .070 | .352 | .276 | .272 |
| 2 hours | .042 | −.772 | −.380 | −.085 | −.963 | .217 | −.680 |
| 4 hours | .152 | .226 | .511 | −.602 | .147 | −.357 | −.180 |
| Time of onset of pain relief | −.040 | −.097 | −.087 | −.144 | −.296 | −.306 | .015 |
| Maximum percent of pain relief | 1.037 | .566 | .535 | −.154 | .328 | .741 | .595 |
| Duration of significant pain relief | .053 | .074 | .166 | .522 | −.249 | −.169 | −.298 |
| Time of greatest change | .018 | .108 | .238 | −.153 | .178 | −.018 | −.001 |
| Increase/no increase in pain | .035 | −.008 | .099 | .133 | −.030 | .042 | .101 |
| Squared multiple correlation | .965 | .886 | .761 | .798 | .489 | .675 | .728 |

judgments and thus increase the likelihood that different results will be obtained at the different centers. The magnitude of such disagreements is assessed in the next section.

## ANALYSIS OF DISAGREEMENT RESULTING FROM DIFFERENT JUDGMENTAL POLICIES

As Lindell (1974) has shown (see also Dawes & Corrigan, 1974), differences in weighting systems do not necessarily produce disagreement. It may be that the intercorrelations among cues are such that investigators with different policies can nevertheless be led to the same conclusions. The analysis of judgment makes it possible to examine the similarities and differences in judgmental policy; however, since each investigator judged different patients, it is not possible to determine a measure of agreement with respect to actual judgments. It is possible, however, to use the above analysis to determine the extent of agreement or disagreement, if (a) each investigator had evaluated every patient in the total sample of 457, and (b) the weights for each investigator (see Table 16.4) were applied with perfect consistency. This determination is accomplished by applying the weights of each physician to the cues for each of the 457 patients and correlating the resulting "predicted judgments" among physicians. The correlations among the investigators' judgments obtained under these conditions measure the agreement produced by judgmental policies and cue intercorrelations (see Table 16.5).

The correlations (ranging from .566 to .944) indicate that there is moderate to

Table 16.5.   Intercorrelations among the Investigators' Judgmental Policies Applied to All Patients

|   | Policy for Investigator | | | | | | |
|---|---|---|---|---|---|---|---|
|   | 1 | 2 | 3 | 4 | 5 | 6 | 7 |
| 1 | 1.000 | .926 | .934 | .814 | .689 | .919 | .863 |
| 2 |   | 1.000 | .944 | .817 | .871 | .835 | .929 |
| 3 |   |   | 1.000 | .804 | .742 | .796 | .867 |
| 4 |   |   |   | 1.000 | .566 | .787 | .728 |
| 5 |   |   |   |   | 1.000 | .703 | .804 |
| 6 |   |   |   |   |   | 1.000 | .771 |
| 7 |   |   |   |   |   |   | 1.000 |

high agreement when these investigators' judgmental policies are applied to these patients (median correlation: .814). There is good general agreement, in spite of considerable disagreement in individual judgmental policy, because some of the cue variables are highly correlated. That is, a *false* agreement occurs as a result of the correlation of cue variables that are differently weighted. For example, the policies of investigators 1 and 2 differed considerably. Investigator 2 placed considerable weight on the report at 2 hours where investigator 1 ignored all cues except the maximum percentage of improvement reported. In spite of this, the application of these policies result in a correlation of .926 because the correlation between maximum percent of improvement and improvement at 2 hours is high (.712).

Such false agreement may or may not have consequences for the evaluation of drug effects. The fact that it can occur, and can be detected by judgment analysis is of considerable importance.

## Analysis of Components of Variation

Although agreement between the judgmental policies of the investigators was relatively high, it was not perfect, and it is possible that the level of disagreement among some investigators was high enough to obscure some treatment effects. In order to separate real differences between treatments from those due to differences in judgmental policy or between the sets of patients, the following analysis was performed:

1. Each physician's policy was applied to the observations on the patients of all other physicians as well as on his own patients. These "predicted effectiveness judgments" $\hat{Y}$ were the dependent variable. They are based on the perfectly consistent application of each physician's policies, and are free from effects due to the inconsistent and unreliable application of judgmental policy.

2. As each investigator's policy was applied to all sets of patients and the latter could also be divided according to the drug each had received, the variance was analyzed by treating policies, drugs, and patients as factors and considering repeated measures over patients (Figure 16.1).

3. The analysis was made separately for two sets of three investigators, those in each set having compared the same three drugs on their patients.

This analysis separates investigator, drug, and patient effects after removing unreliability and answers a number of questions (see Table 16.6).

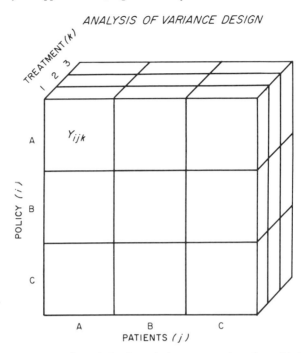

**Figure 16.1.** Analysis of variance design for analyzing treatment, investigators' judgment policies, and patients as independent factors. Each cell contains the predicted effectiveness judgments $Y_{ijk}$ computed by applying the judgment policy of each investigator $i$ to the set of patients $j$ who received treatment $k$. Note that each investigator's judgments are applied to other investigators' patients as well as to his own.

Both analyses show a significant effect for policies: different policies, as expected, cause differences in the mean rating of effectiveness. An individual investigator's preference for the high or low end of the rating scale is maintained when his policy is analyzed. The interaction between policy and patients in both analyses is also significant; the ranking of the mean predicted effectiveness of the policies depends on the set of patients to which the policies are applied. In one of the two analyses, there was a significant effect for patients, indicating that in this sample the predicted effectiveness of treatments differed significantly between groups of patients.

Neither analysis showed a significant main effect for drug treatment nor a significant interaction involving the treatment factor. This is strong evidence that there were no differential treatment effects in either of the two sets examined.

As a check to ensure that evidence of differences between drugs was not inadvertently discarded by the judgmental policy analysis, the residual component

**Table 16.6.    Questions and Appropriate Tests**

| Question | Test |
|---|---|
| 1. Are treatment differences affected when the data is pooled across policies and patients? | Treatment main effect |
| 2. Do different policies cause differences in the mean predicted judgments of different physicians? | Policy main effect |
| 3. Do patients' reports differ? | Patient main effect |
| 4. Are there differences in the effectiveness of the treatments received by the patients of different physicians? | Patient × Treatment interaction |
| 5. Do different policies lead to different conclusions about the relative effectiveness of the treatments? | Policy × Treatment interaction |
| 6. Are the policies influenced by the patients to whom those policies were applied? | Policies × Patients interaction |

of each investigator's judgment was examined. (This component is that part of the investigator's judgment not accounted for by the judgmental analysis and therefore excluded from the analysis of variance.) This check should always be made if these procedures are applied. There was no evidence of treatment effects.

In summary, the following procedure can isolate the components of variation in multicenter clinical trials (or in any situation requiring two or more judges).

1. Analyze the policy of each judge; separate the systematic component of judgment from unreliability.

2. Apply each judge's policy to *all* cases, his own and those of all others, in order to yield predictions of each judge's evaluation of all observations based on the perfectly consistent application of his judgmental policy.

3. Compute intercorrelations among the judges' predictions in order to assess agreement (or false agreement) among the judges with respect to the entire sample of observations.

4. Compute a Policy × Treatments × Sets of observations analysis of variance with the predicted evaluations as the dependent variable in order to separate the systematic component of the judgments into components due to treatment differences, differences between groups, differences in judgmental policies, and interactions between those components.

## CONCLUSION

Replacing the judge does not mean discarding him altogether. When the predicted judgments are substituted for actual judgments, the policy equation is fitted to the cues each judge identified. To develop a single judgment policy that can be applied to all patients in order to eliminate unwanted variation due to inconsistently applied judgmental policies and differences between judges, a joint judgment policy is needed in addition to the relevant cues. Although policy analysis can help, only the judges themselves can *reconcile* their real differences. Once a joint policy has been established, it can be applied to the cue data from *all* centers. Predicted judgments derived from the application of the joint policy to the cue data can then be used in the appropriate statistical test for analysis. Since use of the joint policy eliminates the confounding of judges' judgmental policy and sets of observations, any remaining significant differences between judges must be due to other factors.

In regard to clinical trials, use of the joint policy will have a double effect upon the test of the drug factor. First, sample size can be increased without increasing variability attributable to policy differences between physicians. Second, within-physician judgment error is eliminated, provided that the policy does not change with time. Both effects will increase the power of an experimental design to detect a clinically important, as well as statistically reliable, difference between drugs.

The example used was chosen only to illustrate the potential usefulness of the technique; further work is needed in order to discover the conditions under which treatment differences may be more sensitively detected, and in which the sample size required to detect such differences may be reduced.

## REFERENCES

Bailey, D. E. *Probability and statistics: Models for research.* New York: Wiley, 1971.

Dawes, R. M. and Corrigan, B. Linear models in decision making. *Psychological Bulletin,* 1974, **81,** 95–106.

Lindell, M. Factors affecting measures of linear achievement: Some methodological considerations. Unpublished manuscript, Institute of Behavioral Science, University of Colorado, Program of Research on Human Judgment and Social Interaction, Report No. 167, 1974.

Smith, T. H. A flow chart for policy capturing. Unpublished manuscript, Institute of Behavioral Science, University of Colorado, Program of Research on Human Judgment and Social Interaction, Report No. 147, 1972.

Slovic, P. and Lichtenstein, S. Comparison of Bayesian and regression approaches to the study of information processing in judgment. In L. Rappoport and D. Summers (Eds.), *Human judgment and social interaction.* New York: Holt, Rinehart & Winston, 1973.

# CHAPTER 17

# *Future Research*

C. R. B. JOYCE and KENNETH R. HAMMOND

The final chapter of a book describing the application of a precise theory to a definite practical problem should do more than express pious hopes for the future; it seems necessary to us to criticize the defects of our own methodology. This is not only to anticipate expected and justifiable criticism, but also to present other roads that could be followed in the future.

Our methods are vulnerable on two main grounds—psychological and pharmacological. Many psychologists and psychiatrists may have been surprised and perhaps offended by the apparent neglect of affect. The neglect is more apparent than real, however, for affect *is* allowed to play its part in the studies of interpersonal conflict and interpersonal learning; the subjects are given free rein to express their joy, anger, or annoyance with one another. We have not, however, chosen to *measure* the direction or strength of affect in these circumstances, mainly because nearly every study of interpersonal conflict has done so. Conversely, measurement of cognitive processes has been ignored in virtually every study of interpersonal conflict. We acknowledge, however, that future studies should include measurement of both, and perhaps should include studies of the influence of personality —disappointing as that field has been—as well as of the influence of intelligence, education, and other variables generally included under the rubric of individual differences.

Pharmacologists may also object to our experimental designs because, for example, in acute (single-dose) experiments, the duration of the typical experiment is so long that the blood and brain concentrations of the drug must change markedly during that time; or that in the case of chronic (several day continuous administration) experiments, no attempt was made to correlate effect with the concentrations of drug in blood serum or urine. They might further object that the dose regimes used were extremely narrow and that inference about drug effects from experiments that use only one concentration of a drug is limited at best, as indeed psychologists might object that the individuals studied were samples from rather specialized populations (students, young chronic schizophrenics, etc.).

It is no defense to claim that in these respects ours are no worse than other experiments; or even to claim that they are actually better than most, insofar as they do use a number of different populations, employ wherever possible the classic design principles of random allocation, double-blind, and other controls. Neither is it a defense that few have ever studied to what extent responses of interest in psychopharmacological experiments are disturbed by sampling blood at repeated intervals: experiments in cardiovascular physiology demonstrate clearly that these may in fact be considerable. The risk in deciding not to study such basic correlates was a calculated one. Had our results been overwhelmingly insignificant the cause might well have been one or more of the factors listed above. But significant results from experiments controlled in the ways described indicate that the observed events were real, and that there is a serious phenomenon to account for. So far from lacking the appropriate kind of control, the work has in fact introduced at least one major new methodological concept of wide potential application (see Chapter 13 by Gillis): the establishment as a standard of clinically defined adequate therapeutic regime enables other objectively or subjectively measured drug effects to be compared across patients. Heretofore, differences in regime have presented a problem to experimental investigators, whose approach to the patient under treatment is often less realistic than that of the patient himself. To insist on a standardized regime for all patients being investigated is surely even less reasonable than to insist that patients on identical regimes also be comparable in all other possible ways—yet the latter is rightly held to be unrealistic though the former is almost always considered essential.

Irrespective of the reader's satisfaction or dissatisfaction with the studies reported in this book, we can all agree on the need for more and better research regarding the effects of psychoactive drugs on social judgment. The present lack of knowledge about the effects of centrally active drugs on intellectual processes in general, and interpersonal learning and interpersonal conflict arising from different judgment policies in particular, has important implications for the future. However useful present drugs may be for sedating, tranquilizing, and removing or reducing phobias and hallucinations for the troubled patient, if our aim is to improve cognitive functioning in persons who suffer a deficit in that regard, much more needs to be done. Indeed, a great deal needs to be done if a physician is to be able to make an informed choice of medication. Our belief is that the kind of research described here will eventually help the physician to choose the drug with the least social toxicity. That choice will be particularly important if clinical evidence continues to suggest that several psychoactive drugs are of equal help with regard to symptom alleviation, while experimental research on social judgment shows that these drugs produce differential impairment of cognitive function. Therein lies the need for the research in the future. The continuation of research on the effects of psychoactive drugs on social judgment should lead to the discovery of drugs that *enhance* the social judgment of those whose impaired judgment resulted in their hospitalization.

Neither traditional psychopharmacological studies nor those reported here indicate that "normal" cognitive functions are improved by psychoactive drugs, although theoretically it should be possible to improve the cognitive competence of the normal adult, as well as that of the disturbed, while interfering as little as possible with his social functioning. It also should be possible to improve social function with minimal interference to individual behavior. The very existence of these possibilities is bound to challenge scientists to turn them into realities. Therefore, society will eventually have to ask itself what efforts to normalize or idealize (supernormalize) are really desirable and really needed, and if the benefit would exceed the cost. There seems little doubt that this question will soon become a public issue, probably within the present decade.

The pressure for better, that is, wiser, judgments in matters of social policy will also increase, particularly if shortages of food, water, and energy increase as expected, and as it becomes more apparent that the source of all social policies is human judgment. But there is little reason for the expectation that human judgment as it now functions will be adequate for coping with the complexity that worldwide interdependence brings. It is not difficult to create a laboratory task to defeat the best cognitive effort any individual or group can muster; judgment tasks in the world outside the laboratory are clearly still more difficult. Moreover, the present confusion, chaos, and defeat in the social process arising from the inadequacy of past and present social policies also give reason to believe that man's cognitive competence is insufficient to cope with the future policy-making tasks that confront him. In short, it seems likely to us that there will be a steady pressure to allow, even to encourage, attempts at improving man's cognitive competence because the need for survival will demand it.

The fact that none of the drugs we have so far studied shows that interpersonal learning is improved above the placebo level does not mean that no such drugs exist or will be discovered. The number studied has been small, the techniques used have been specialized and may not have been the most sensitive or appropriate. Only those who believe that the intellect of the typical man or woman is incapable of improvement are likely to think that the answers to such questions are not worth exploring.

We believe that the need to study the effect of drugs on personal interaction, and the reverse, will grow in importance for what may be termed tactical day-by-day reasons as well as those of long-term survival strategy. On purely statistical grounds the probability at an encounter between no more than two people that one of them will have taken at least one drug (including alcohol) is at present between 50 and 80%; and that *both* will have done so is between 6 and 16%. If present trends continue, these proportions will increase. Although it has been predicted that "Most Americans will continue to prefer mild to strong intoxicants, legal to illegal drugs, social to solitary pursuit of pleasure, and the loosening of inhibitions to the profound spiritual experience [Newitt, Singer, & Kahn, 1971, p. 114]," the consequences of even this legal, social, disinhibiting use of mild substances to family, business, and other group decision-making situations remains for the moment almost totally unexplored. The use of drugs for emotional disturbances (both on a self-medicating and physician-ordered basis) is certainly growing at present. Whether or not this use is already excessive is (perhaps surprisingly to some) still a matter of dispute (Joyce, 1974).

Even if the trends were to remain stationary, however, we would still need to know how drugs influence judgments *of* the drugged, *about* the drugged, and arising from the *interaction* of the drugged with others. How much of our present legislation and other political activity represents interaction modified by such means? Is it better or worse for having been initiated in smoke-filled rooms and wine-filled brains? How many of our future, perhaps present, legislators are experienced users of social drugs other than alcohol and tobacco, and how much difference does this make to their decisions on matters other than drugs?

We began this study with the belief that scientific progress comes with the continual interaction of theory, method, and data, and we therefore organized the work in this book to reflect that interaction. We conclude with the hope that the reader shares our belief, and finds that we were faithful to our aims.

**REFERENCES**

Joyce, C. R. B. Who does what to whom and why? In M. Balter (Ed.), *Proceedings of the conference on anxiolytic drugs*. Rockville, Md.: National Institutes of Mental Health 1974.

Newitt, J., Singer, M., and Kahn, H. Some speculations on U.S. drug use. *Journal of Social Issues*, 1971, **27**, (3), 107–122.

# Author Index

# Subject Index